Foundations for Paramedic Practice

A Theoretical Perspective

Amanda Blaber

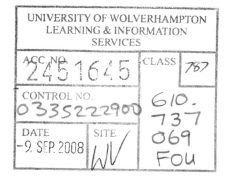

Open University Press

Open University Press
McGraw-Hill Education
McGraw-Hill House
Shoppenhangers Road
Maidenhead
Berkshire
England
SL6 2QL

email: enquiries@openup.co.uk
world wide web: www.openup.co.uk

and
Two Penn Plaza
New York, NY 10121–2289, USA

First published 2008

A catalogue record of this book is available from the British Library

ISBN13: 978 0 335 22289 6 (pb)   978 0 335 22290 2 (hb)
ISBN10: 0 335 22289 7 (pb)   0 335 22290 0 (hb)

Library of Congress Cataloging-in-Publication Data
CIP data has been applied for

Typeset by RefineCatch Limited, Bungay, Suffolk
Printed in Great Britain by Bell and Bain Ltd., Glasgow

Fictitious names of companies, products, people, characters and/or data that
may be used herein (in case studies or in examples) are not intended to
represent any real individual, company, product or event.

The **McGraw-Hill** Companies

For all of our friends and family, past and present

Contents

List of contributors

Amanda Blaber
Teaching Fellow
PG (Dip)Ed, MSc Sociology of Health and Welfare, BSc (Hons) Health and Community Studies, Dip HE (Accident & Emergency), RGN
Department of Acute and Continuing Care, School of Health and Social Care, University of Greenwich

Amanda has a background in acute medical and emergency care nursing. This area of expertise naturally lends itself to partnerships and teamwork with ambulance service colleagues. After 12 years and working at the level of Senior Sister, Amanda decided to accept the new challenge of higher education. Whilst working at the University of Hertfordshire, Amanda taught student nurses and paramedics, on both pre- and post-qualifying pathways. After moving to the University of Greenwich in 2003, Amanda led the curriculum development with the London Ambulance Service to achieve validation of the Foundation Degree (FdSc) in 2006. Amanda believes that an understanding of subject specialisms such as sociology and psychology is vital to the development of the twenty-first-century paramedic and is the reason for this book being written. Amanda believes that this holistic approach to patient care can impact on the brief but vital periods of time spent with patients and improve the quality of care provided.

Alison Cork
Senior Lecturer
MA HE, BSc (Hons), RN
Department of Acute and Continuing Care, School of Health and Social Care, University of Greenwich

Alison qualified as a nurse in 1989 and worked in the specialism of Emergency Care for 15 years. Having risen through the ranks to Senior Sister, Alison chose to follow a path into education, both in clinical practice and for the last three years in a higher education setting, in both nursing and paramedic practice. Alison finds it very rewarding to see the personal and professional growth of the students and helping them on their way to challenging, yet satisfying careers.

Steve Cowland
Training Officer
BSc, PGCE, paramedic, IHCD driving tutor
Bromley Education and Development Centre, London Ambulance Service NHS Trust

Steve joined the London Ambulance Service in 1984. He has been a paramedic since 1991 and now works as an ambulance tutor. He has been involved with higher education programmes both as a student undertaking his BSc (Hons) Paramedic Science, completed in 2004, and as a teacher and a link tutor for students undertaking the FdSc Paramedic Science at the University of Greenwich. Steve successfully completed his postgraduate diploma in Higher Education in 2008.

Brian Craggs
Education Centre Manager at Bromley Ambulance Education and Development Centre
BSc (Hons), paramedic, IHCD driving tutor, IHCD Directing staff, IHCD/Edexcel external verifier
London Ambulance Service (LAS) NHS Trust
Currently acting Clinical Education Manager at Education and Development Headquarters, Fulham, London

Brian joined the LAS in 1975 and worked at Westminster for nine years, where he gained experience during the many bombing incidents in the 1970s and 1980s. Brian worked on the HEMS air ambulance during its first year of operation in London. In 1984, he qualified as an Institute of Health Care Development (IHCD) tutor and moved into the Training Department. Brian graduated from the University of Hertfordshire as a member of the first part-time route cohort, BSc (Hons) Paramedic Science in 2000.

Rachael Donohoe
Head of Clinical Audit and Research
PhD, BSc (Hons)
London Ambulance Service NHS Trust

Rachael has a long track record in managing large-scale health-related research projects and is seen as a leading expert in clinical audit. Since joining the London Ambulance Service NHS Trust as Head of Clinical Audit and Research, Rachael has been involved in numerous ground-breaking pre-hospital research projects and led the way in promoting clinical audit within the ambulance service. Her involvement in clinical audit and research, both within the wider NHS and with external international partners, has led to changes to practice and patient care and influenced national pre-hospital clinical guidelines. In light of her commitment to pre-hospital audit and research, she was recently granted honorary research fellow status at Kingston University and St George's Medical School. She is also Chair of the South of England Ambulance Clinical Audit Group, which steers the development of clinical audit at a regional level.

Bob Fellows
Education Development Manager
BSc Paramedic Science (UH), PGCE (UH)
London Ambulance Service NHS Trust

Bob joined the London Ambulance Service in 1980 after four years as a gardener/nurseryman for the London Borough of Brent. Bob has held several roles, but most related to education and organizational development. He has been involved in most clinical situations that are the norm for an ambulance person, plus a few that are distinctly not normal, including three major incidents, the last being in July 2005 at Edgware Road tube station.

Bob is privileged to be Chairperson of the British Paramedic Association and has spent the past 15 months editing a textbook for paramedics called *Nancy Caroline's Emergency Care in the Streets*.

Graham Harris
Training Officer
BSc, PGCE, Chartered MCIPD, AASI, Advanced BTec MHPE, paramedic Bromley Education and Development Centre, London Ambulance Service NHS Trust

Graham has 23 years' experience with the London Ambulance Service, 17 of these as a paramedic and 19 years as an ambulance tutor. He has been involved with higher education programmes for a decade, both as a student undertaking his BSc Paramedic Science and presently completing his MSc in Education and Management, and as a link tutor for students undertaking the FdSc Paramedic Science at the University of Greenwich.

Paul Street
Teaching Fellow
EdD, MSc, PGDE, BSc (Hons), DipN (Lond), RGN, EN
Department of Acute and Continuing Care, School of Health and Social Care, University of Greenwich

Paul has a broad nursing background in clinical practice, education and practice development. He started as an enrolled nurse in general surgery in 1982. Before becoming a Teaching Fellow/Skills Coordinator he worked clinically in medical and surgical areas, HIV and AIDS areas, practice development and pre-registration nursing education. He passionately believes that communication and interpersonal skills lie at the heart of all healthcare practice.

Jackie Whitnell
Senior Lecturer
PG (Dip) HE, MA Sociology of Health and Welfare, BSc (Hons) Psychology, CPHSN (HV), RSCN, RGN, EN
Department of Family Care and Mental Health, School of Health and Social Care, University of Greenwich

Jackie has a 28-year history of working within the NHS. Her early career included theatre and intensive care nursing. She has also given 18 years to children's services, as a sick children's nurse and then in primary care as a health visitor. Jackie has a BSc (Hons) in psychology, and a Masters (MA) in sociology, which she believes has led to a more comprehensive understanding of psychology, sociology and child development. Jackie has been working as a lecturer since 2002. She has taught abnormal and developmental psychology and aspects of child health to student nurses and paramedics both at the University of Hertfordshire and the University of Greenwich. Jackie is committed to educating students in her chosen topic areas and is always enthusiastic in the delivery of her teaching sessions.

Acknowledgements

Thanks to all the contributors, whose hard work has made this project possible.

Introduction

There is no shortage of textbooks for ambulance clinicians that discuss the practical aspects of the role. The *translation* of these texts to the British market has occurred (Caroline 2007), but there are far fewer texts relating to the theoretical aspects encompassed within a paramedic's role. Having been involved in the education of ambulance personnel and healthcare professionals over the last seven years, either qualified technicians and paramedics, student paramedics or students of allied health professions, I have observed that many students found the more theoretical aspects of study much more difficult than the *doing* aspects of their role. Indeed, there are numerous texts that focus upon the physical sciences, anatomy and physiology and technical procedures. This book aims to introduce some of the main social science (and other related) theoretical subjects that a student will be required to study when undertaking either a full-time pre registration or post-qualifying part-time programme. You will not find anatomy, physiology, bioscience or pharmacology covered within this text, as it can be broadly categorized as covering the psycho-social science aspects of any higher education paramedic curriculum. This was a deliberate choice, as there are many core texts covering such aspects, that are highly pertinent to paramedic education available within the United Kingdom at this time.

Within this book, the emphasis is very much on 'introduction' to these subjects; each chapter contains full referencing and some suggested reading so that you can access more specific texts or websites if you wish to investigate further. This book is by no means an *all you need to know* text; it should be used in conjunction with other more specific textbooks/articles/websites. Each chapter discusses the relevance of the chapter to the ambulance clinician. It is intended to be a 'foundation' text, suitable for new recruits to the paramedic profession or existing qualified clinicians and healthcare professionals who are entering higher education for the first time. It is hoped the text will provide a basis on which students can build their knowledge and education and link the theoretical concepts to their clinical role. It is suggested that students also consult a study skills book, in order to develop study and writing skills, as it is highly likely that they will be required to produce written work for many assessments. There are many suitable texts available (which is why this text does not include study skills): ask the advice of programme or course leaders.

All the contributors are either qualified, experienced paramedics themselves and/or work for ambulance NHS Trusts in education/quality roles, or are experienced healthcare professionals and academics with experience of teaching student paramedics and other allied health professionals. The choice of contributors has been deliberate, as they have been required to include *stop and think* points that directly relate to the ambulance clinician's role. It is hoped that the stop and think sections will provoke students to think about things in a different way, question their actions and generate discussion with colleagues. There are also *link to* prompts that have been included to highlight how the various chapters (or sections of chapters) relate to one another, enhancing the opportunity for the reader to understand the links between the various theoretical perspectives. In many of the chapters there are press extracts; these serve to explain the points made within the chapter, which the reader might find quite abstract concepts on a first read. It is hoped that the reader finds these press extracts interesting and that they support and help to explain the theoretical concept that is being discussed. It is important that the text is relevant to the reader, so the choice of contributors with credibility in their own subject area and experience of teaching/ working with ambulance clinicians has ensured that relevance is paramount and examples used are pre-hospital specific.

The aim of this book is to underpin practice and link the reader's ways of working to the extremely important theory base. If the reader is successful and this aim is achieved, it will serve to promote professionalism in the student's day-to-day working life. As readers may be aware, 77 per cent of patients/clients from emergency calls are transported to the hospital (ONS 2005). The remaining 23 per cent are patients/ clients that are likely to be treated at home or 'on scene'. Figures from the Department of Health (2005) suggest that half of the 77 per cent who are transported to hospital could be treated at the scene or in their own homes. Therefore, the essential understanding of theory and practice together provides clinicians with the knowledge to do justice to their role, extend their skills, and provide appropriate, informed and professional care to patients.

References

Caroline, N. (2007) *Emergency Care on the Streets*. London: Jones and Bartlett Publishers.

Department of Health (2005) *Taking Healthcare to the Patient: Transforming NHS Ambulance Services*. London: DoH.

NHS Confederation (2007) *NHS Ambulance Services . . . More Than Just Patient Transport*. London: NHS Confederation.

Office for National Statistics (2005) *National Statistics: Ambulance Services 2004/2005*. London: ONS.

1

Consideration of history
Brian Craggs and Amanda Blaber

Topics covered:

- Introduction
- Why is this relevant?
- Brief history of the National Health Service (NHS)
- Historical development of the ambulance service in the United Kingdom
- Modernization of ambulance services
- Professional registration and regulation
- Conclusion
- Chapter key points
- References, suggested reading and useful websites

Introduction

The NHS has distinct differences from any other health service anywhere in the world. It is important for any healthcare professional to have an understanding of how the NHS developed and the circumstances surrounding its emergence. An appreciation of the planning, main figures and the battles fought to achieve the service that we are part of today is important to provide us all with a sense of history and to uphold the intended principles of the NHS. Today, the NHS cares for over one million patients every 36 hours (NHS Confederation 2007a). The sheer scale of the NHS is remarkable and has a fascinating historical development. As with any organization of this magnitude, it does not always get everything right; the consequences of mistakes in the NHS can be catastrophic and sometimes the difference between life and death.

Why is this relevant?

The development of ambulance services is one aspect of NHS provision today; the emergence of ambulance services as a main provider of care to the population is interesting. The NHS is an expanding organization: since 2000 the number of frontline staff has risen by 21 per cent. This rise includes a 21 per cent increase in doctors, 25 per cent increase in nurses and 17 per cent increase in ambulance staff (NHS Confederation 2007b). An understanding of developments in education, role development and professionalization are important to any student or qualified practitioner, in order that they can impact on the future of their profession.

Brief history of the National Health Service (NHS)

On 5 July 1948, a date of significant importance to all residents of the United Kingdom (UK), the National Health Service was launched. Its aim was to provide people in need with a range of health services. The history of the inception of the NHS is an interesting mix of legislation, power, negotiation and collaboration. In order to trace a brief overview of events leading to 1948, it is perhaps wise to discuss events up to one hundred years before.

Hospitals date back to medieval times: St Bartholomew's and St Thomas's in London were formed in 1123 and 1215 respectively, by religious foundations. It was not until the thirteenth century that further building of hospitals occurred. Records show that even this early, three distinct types of doctor emerged:

- physicians – elite doctors with university-based training;
- barber-surgeons – a guild-organized apprenticeship;
- apothecaries – developed from shopkeepers who provided basic medical care and administered drugs. The original 'general practitioner' (GP).

Most hospitals at this time had religious connections, so the dissolution of the monasteries by Henry VIII in the sixteenth century had a huge impact on their survival. Within London, only St Bartholomew's, St Thomas's and the Bethlem survived this period of history. Further hospital building did not occur until the eighteenth century.

It is also interesting to note that until the eighteenth century childbirth remained the domain of midwives and women only. Edwin Chadwick championed the public health movement and campaigned for the improvement in adequate water supplies and sewerage systems (Ham 2004). In 1848 the Public Health Act led to further Acts and eventual appointment of a medical officer for health in 1872. The Medical Act of 1858 aimed to regulate medicine and at this time a national register of qualified medical practitioners was established.

Once hospitals had been built, the nineteenth century saw more radical specialization of doctors and with them developed specialist hospitals, many of which are still evident today. Prior to the second half of the nineteenth century, workhouses had provided relief and care for the poor, as the voluntary hospitals were more concerned with the acutely ill (perhaps as a result of doctors specializing) and refused admission to the more chronically ill and those with infectious disease. Consequently, work-houses were often overcrowded and were the source of many outbreaks of illness.

> **Stop and think** – What are the specialist hospitals in your region? Do you know the history of them?

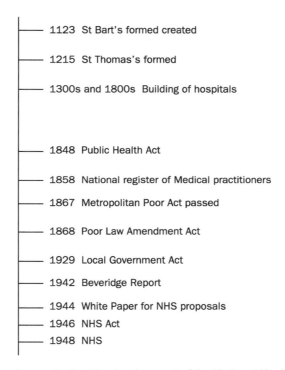

1123 St Bart's formed created

1215 St Thomas's formed

1300s and 1800s Building of hospitals

1848 Public Health Act

1858 National register of Medical practitioners

1867 Metropolitan Poor Act passed

1868 Poor Law Amendment Act

1929 Local Government Act

1942 Beveridge Report

1944 White Paper for NHS proposals

1946 NHS Act

1948 NHS

Figure 1.1 Timeline demonstrating the development of the National Health Service

In 1867 the Metropolitan Poor Act was passed and public infirmaries were created, separate to the existing workhouses. This was made law first in London and then across the country through the 1868 Poor Law Amendment Act. This is a key moment in English social history, as it was the first time the state had accepted its duty to provide hospitals for the poor (Ham 2004). Further steps towards today's NHS were made with the passing of the 1929 Local Government Act. This Act superseded the Poor Law and made local authorities responsible for workhouses and infirmaries, as with other public services, all under the control of medical officers of health. The latter end of the nineteenth century also saw a more marked separation of community services, led by GPs and hospital-based specialists.

The outbreak of the Second World War led to public hospitals with a wide range of general and specialist services joining the voluntary hospitals in the Emergency

Medical Service (EMS). This enabled coordination of services and resources to support the war effort. The framework for administration of hospitals after the war was taken from the regional organization of the EMS. At this time the government announced plans to develop a National *Hospital* Service. In 1942 the Beveridge Report on Social Insurance and Allied Services recommended extension of the social security system and other reforms. In addition, proposals for a National *Health* Service were included, adding weight to the government's proposals.

Link to Chapter 13, Social policy, for definitions and explanations of White and Green Papers

A White Paper in 1944 outlining NHS proposals was made, with the NHS Act following in 1946 and the creation of the service in 1948. The name Aneurin Bevan (Labour government Minister for Health after election victory in 1945) is synonymous with the creation of the NHS and he was involved in prolonged negotiations with the medical profession prior to 1948. Ham (2004: 14) states that the medical profession fought strongly for its own objectives, namely:

- retention of the independent contractor system for GPs;
- the option of private practice and access to pay beds in NHS hospitals for hospital consultants;
- a system of distinction awards for consultants, carrying with it large increases in salary for those receiving awards;
- a major role in the administration of the Service at all levels;
- success in resisting local government control.

Bevan had in fact divided hospital doctors (by providing financial incentives) from their GP colleagues (he reduced their power and isolated them), and in doing so reduced the total power wielded by the medical profession. The GPs did eventually achieve many of their aims, though. Had Bevan not chosen to adopt this approach, maybe the process of establishing the NHS would have taken even longer. Many doctors wanted the NHS to provide for only 90 per cent of the population. Bevan personally persuaded the profession that the service should be totally inclusive: we can see that he succeeded. Since its inception, the NHS has undergone many changes, but the way it is funded, mainly out of general taxation with insurance contributions only making up a small part of the total money required, is the same today as Bevan and other influential colleagues had planned prior to 1948. Many of the proposed keystones of the NHS still remain today.

Knowing the background to the processes involved in the creation of the NHS should enable ambulance clinicians to have more understanding of the history of the service within which they work. Exploring history very often provides explanations of the way things are today, so it is also important to explore the history of the ambulance service.

Historical development of the ambulance service in the United Kingdom

Worldwide

As an emergency service, the ambulance service is relatively young, being pre-dated by fire and police services by many years. The use of dedicated ambulance transport as a means of providing some clinical care in the field and transporting the injured to a place for further treatment can be traced back to the Napoleonic era when in 1793 Dominique-Jean Larrey (1766–1842), a bright young surgeon in Bonaparte's army, first utilized light horse-drawn carts as 'mobile field hospitals', to move and treat the injured on the battlefield. The corps of nurses and surgeons who operated this early system became known as 'ambulance volante', meaning flying ambulance (Robertson-Steel 2005). This and other developments earned Larrey favour with the Emperor Napoleon who promoted him to Surgeon-in-Chief of his armies and later made him a baron. Since then the development of ambulance services worldwide has been considerable and varied, with different systems under the direction of different authorities.

United Kingdom (UK)

In the UK, ambulance service provision developed from early police-operated hand litters and the Metropolitan Asylums Board horse-drawn fever ambulances of the 1860s, through the two World Wars and motorization of vehicles, with relatively little change in the level of care provided by its operatives. Though gaining importance during this time, ambulance work was regarded as little more than manual labour, with minimal clinical control and regulation. About one hundred years on from those 1860s horse-drawn vehicles came the first real attempt at providing guidelines for the regulation of ambulance service provision in the UK. The Millar report (Ministry of Health 1966) laid down recommendations for equipment and minimum acceptable levels of training and equipment for the, then, County Council-run ambulance services. Prior to this, the training consisted of no more than a civil defence corps first aid course.

1970s to present day

It was only comparatively recently that the medicalization process began and in 1974 responsibility for the UK ambulance service was transferred to the National Health Service. From then to the present day there has been an unprecedented expansion in 'out-of-hospital' care delivery, with the advent of limited advanced training (intubation and infusion) in the early 1970s, through the initial vestiges and development of advanced cardiac life support with defibrillators, trauma care and paramedics of the 1980s. The 1990s brought 'Trust' status to ambulance services and saw the continued development of paramedic practice. As a result of clinical audit and research, the devolution of some of the previously 'reserved skills' to be practised by ambulance technicians was enabled.

Link to clinical audit part of Chapter 4, pages 43–8 for more detail about the role and importance of clinical audit. Link to Chapter 16 to explore the purpose and value of keeping up-to-date as a registered paramedic practitioner.

Such interventions as cardiac defibrillation, nebulization therapy and the parenteral administration of certain prescription-only medicines entered the domain of the technician. This represented a significant step in the development of evidence-based clinical practice and may be perceived as a major landmark in the professionalization of the UK ambulance service. The latter part of the 1990s bore several government publications aimed at developing the Health Service in general and ambulance services in particular.

Link to Chapter 4, pages 48–55, for explanation on the role of evidence-based practice and its influence on the development of the paramedic profession.

Modernization of ambulance services

The health service circular entitled *Modernisation of Ambulance Services* (NHS Executive 1999) clearly sets out the government's view that 'quality care should be at the heart of the National Health Service'. It places ambulance services at the forefront of 'the new NHS modernization programme' (UK Parliament 1997), aiming to ensure that they perform a key role in the development of quality systems encompassing many areas of healthcare delivery. It emphasizes the importance of national standards to ensure consistent, high-quality care as specified in 'a first class service' (NHS Executive 1998).

Link to Chapter 4, pages 39–43, to explore what these phrases mean in terms of clinical governance and how they shape paramedic practice.

An example of the influence of national standards

Major emphasis was placed on the National Service Framework (NSF) for Coronary Heart Disease (NHS Executive 2000) and many ambulance services have responded as directed by undertaking pre-hospital thrombolysis for those patients suitably diagnosed. Others, notably London, have embarked on a programme of alliance with hospitals offering primary angioplasty as the gold standard intervention for confirmed myocardial infarction (MI). In either system, the ambulance crew are able to make the diagnosis of MI using a 12-lead electrocardiogram (ECG) and other key factors. With this system, instead of giving a thrombolytic drug, the crew can rapidly transport the patient to one of the cardiac catheterization laboratories in the capital. This practice has produced impressive results in terms of patient outcome and reduced aftercare and carries less risk than that of primary thrombolysis.

Training

UK ambulance services currently conform to training standards as laid down by the Institute of Health Care Development (IHCD). This means that both paramedic and ambulance technician training follow an agreed strategy which is supported by a paramedic steering group composed of local clinicians. For many years the national ambulance service has fulfilled its basic role of 'treat and transport'; it has now become appropriate to consider modifications in thinking and extend the role of the paramedic to that of a 'practitioner'.

Education and the future

A report published in January 2000 by the Joint Royal Colleges Ambulance Liaison Committee (JRCALC) and the Ambulance Service Association (ASA) examined the future role and education of paramedic ambulance service personnel. The opening sentence in the report stated that 'Emergency pre-hospital care can have a profound influence on morbidity and mortality of those critically ill or injured' (JRCALC 2000: 3). It supports the concept of developing the role of the paramedic and envisages 'a health care professional with a degree, and commitment to long term development of skills and education' (JRCALC 2000: 7). The committee suggested an appropriate generic title for this professional as 'Practitioner in Emergency Care' (PEC). This concept has already been pursued by many ambulance Trusts throughout the country, resulting in partnerships with universities, facilitating degree courses for paramedics. This is widely regarded as a considerable step towards fulfilling this role, though the more widely used title seems to be emergency care practitioner or ECP, which also embraces nurses and other generic healthcare workers.

Professional registration and regulation

This, coupled with the advent of professional paramedic registration with the Council for Professions Supplementary to Medicine and latterly the Health Professions Council (HPC), has the effect of placing paramedics in the forefront of emergency care, with the ability to practise flexibly in a variety of primary care areas and have an even greater influence on the morbidity and mortality of the critically ill or injured. It was required that the HPC should liaise with a professional body for each of the practitioner groups on the register; all except the ambulance service had such a body. As a result of this, in 2001 the British Paramedic Association (BPA) was formed, as the representative professional body for paramedics.

Conclusion

In its publication *Taking Healthcare to the Patient: Transforming NHS Ambulance Services* (DoH 2005: 50 point E8), the Department of Health recommends that 'Ambulance clinicians should be equipped with a greater range of competencies that enable them to assess, treat, refer, or discharge an increasing number of patients and meet quality requirements for urgent care'. This supports the inevitable movement of ambulance education towards partnerships with higher education institutes. Such partnerships have begun the development of the role of the emergency care practitioner and have resulted in attractive alternative pathways to paramedic practice. No longer is it the sole domain of the ambulance service under the verification of the IHCD to train paramedics. Ambulance NHS Trusts are developing numerous programmes, at varying academic levels, with higher education institutes, in response to their individual service requirements for their regions. Thus ambulance service education has progressed into the twenty-first century with greater integration into university schemes across a wide spectrum of related subjects.

Link to Chapter 13 to read about policy that is shaping future practice.

Chapter key points

- In order to appreciate health care within twenty-first-century Britain an understanding of health care in Britain prior to the NHS is important.
- The development of ambulance services within the UK is of interest to ambulance clinicians and may help explain some of the practice unique to the service today.
- The chapter discusses the future developments of the ambulance service and provides the reader with a clear idea of future developments.

References and suggested reading

Audit Commission (1998) *A Life in the Fast Lane: Value for Money in Emergency Ambulance Services*. London: Audit Commission/HMSO.

DoH (Department of Health) (2005) *Taking Healthcare to the Patient: Transforming NHS Ambulance Services*. UK: DoH Publications.

Ham, C. (2004) *Health Policy in Britain*, 5th edn. Basingstoke: Palgrave Macmillan.

Joint Royal Colleges Ambulance Liaison Committee (2000) *The Future Role and Education of Paramedic Ambulance Service Personnel*. London: JRCALC.

Ministry of Health, Scottish Home and Health Department (1966) *Report by the Working Party on Ambulance Training and Equipment* (Millar Report). *Part 1: Training*. London: HMSO.

National Health Service Executive (1998) *A First Class Service*, Health Service Circular 1998/113. London: NHS Executive.

National Health Service Executive (1999) *Modernisation of Ambulance Services*. Health Service Circular 1999/091. London: NHS Executive.

National Health Service Executive (2000) *National Service Framework for Coronary Heart Disease: Modern Standards and Service Models*. London: NHS Executive.

NHS Confederation (2007a) *Key Statistics on the NHS*. London: NHS Confederation.

NHS Confederation (2007b) *NHS Ambulance Services . . . More Than Just Patient Transport*. London: NHS Confederation.

Robertson-Steel, I. (2005) Evolution of triage systems, *Emergency Medicine Journal*, 23: 154–5.

United Kingdom Parliament (1997) *The New NHS: Modern, Dependable*, Cm 3807. London: HMSO.

United Kingdom Parliament (1999) *Health Act*. London: The Stationery Office.

Useful websites

NHS History: www.nhshistory.net
NHS Confederation: www.nhsconfed.org
NHS Connecting for Health: www.nhs.uk

2

Ethics and law for the paramedic
Graham Harris and Steve Cowland

Topics covered:

- Introduction
- Why is this relevant?
- Confidentiality and data protection
- Accountability
- Health Profession Council practice committees
- Consent
- Conclusion
- Chapter key points
- References and suggested reading

Introduction

Public regard for paramedics and ambulance clinicians remains high. The clinical performance of these health professionals has undergone enormous change in the past two decades, culminating in the professional registration of paramedics in July 2003 (HPC 2003). The advances in clinical practice and professional standards for paramedics require them to adhere to the standards prescribed by their registrant body, the Health Professions Council (HPC). These standards incorporate the principles of conduct, performance and ethics. However, other areas within paramedic practice, such as driving, still require compliance with road traffic law and the exemptions therein (for example those provided to emergency personnel responding to an emergency call under the Road Traffic Act 1988). Therefore, paramedics are required to adhere to a wide array of professional standards and law to ensure that they provide the optimal paramedic practice delivery.

Why is this relevant?

Paramedics meet people often in extremely difficult and distressing personal circumstances and at critical times in their lives. Patients and families are vulnerable during these moments, so it is critical that ambulance clinicians have an understanding of key ethical issues they are most likely to meet on an everyday basis. Exploring some of these issues may prepare clinicians for dilemmas they may encounter. Due to the nature of the clinician's role, ethical issues across the lifespan also require examination. No text can prepare the reader for all eventualities, but a discussion of the key ethical issues is vital for safe, competent and professional practice.

Confidentiality and data protection

The NHS Code of Practice, *Confidentiality* (DoH 2003a:11), clearly defines a duty of confidence as:

> when one person discloses information to another e.g. patient to clinician in circumstances where it is reasonable to expect that the information will be held in confidence. It is:
>
> a.   A legal obligation that is derived from case law;
> b.   A requirement established within professional codes of conduct; and
> c.   Must be included within NHS employment contracts as specific requirement linked to disciplinary procedures.

The Health Professions Council (2003: 6) states that 'You must treat information about patients, clients or users as confidential and use it only for the purpose for which it was given. You must not knowingly release any personal or confidential information to anyone who is not entitled to it, and you should check that people who ask for information are entitled to it.' The *UK Ambulance Service Clinical Practice Guidelines* (JRCALC 2006) provide guidance concerning the ethical issue of confidentiality. Practitioners should ensure that information regarding their patient is recorded clearly and precisely so that the patient's care pathway is processed without error.

Case study

A patient complains to an ambulance NHS Trust about her treatment en route to hospital. During the investigation, the patient's report form is examined. Among other details the investigator sees the following: Impression PVD.

    The clinician who wrote the form is called upon to explain her treatment. The investigator asks what was wrong with the patient. The clinician cannot understand this question, as it is clear to her that PVD is an abbreviation she uses for per vaginal discharge. The investigator makes it clear that his interpretation of PVD is peripheral vascular disease.

The above case study highlights the importance of trying not to use abbreviations on official documentation, as this can be misunderstood.

Stop and think – Have you ever had to answer a complaint as a result of poor recording/documentation of a patient's care? Think about what may influence your ability to follow these documentation guidelines. What strategies could you use to ensure your documentation is clear and precise?

In order to protect patient information the guidelines provide five essential steps to ensure compliance with the relevant standards of confidentiality. See Box 2.1.

Box 2.1 Five essential steps to ensure compliance with standards of confidentiality (JRCALC 2006)

1. Record patient information concisely and accurately.
2. Keep patient information physically secure.
3. Follow guidance before disclosing any patient information.
4. Conform to best practice.
5. Anonymize information where possible.

The principles outlined in Box 2.1 need to be supported by ambulance service policies and procedures that incorporate the ethos of the Data Protection Act (HMSO 1998), which describes the processes for obtaining, recording, holding, using and sharing information.

The issue of confidentiality is one that requires careful management by paramedics. When dealing with the public, healthcare professionals and other professional bodies, there is a potential for information to be leaked about patients and their treatment. It is easy at the scene of an emergency call to declare information about a patient that may be overheard by members of the public. Patient records present another risk to patient confidentiality. Forms completed by paramedics with respect to patient treatment and details must be recorded as accurately as possible and be protected from viewing by those not entitled to do so. Safe storage and disposal of these forms is also a requirement of the Data Protection Act (1998) and various ambulance service policies and procedures should reflect this requirement.

Stop and think – Have you observed colleagues try to maintain patient confidentiality in public places during an emergency? Think about the strategies you can use to try and maintain confidentiality in emergency situations. Also think about the possible consequences of ignoring the importance of trying to maintain confidentiality.

The relationship between healthcare professionals and their patients has always been considered especially significant with regard to disclosure of information. Much of the information given to the paramedic practitioner is often of a sensitive nature and there is an expectation that this information will not be passed onto others without the consent of the individual concerned. The confidentiality model (see Figure 2.1) advocated by the Department of Health (2003a: 10) may help to remind paramedics of their main responsibilities regarding patient confidentiality.

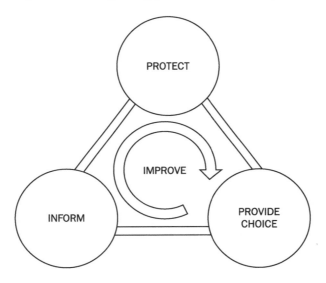

a. PROTECT – look after the patient's information;
b. INFORM – ensure that patients are aware of how their information is used;
c. PROVIDE CHOICE – allow patients to decide whether their information can be disclosed or used in particular ways. To support these three requirements, there is a fourth:
d. IMPROVE – always look for better ways to protect, inform and provide choice.

Figure 2.1 The confidentiality model
Source: DoH (2003a: 10)

This model will naturally involve paramedics in other aspects of quality monitoring, such as clinical audit, in order to establish ways to improve their own and others' professional practice.

Link to Chapter 4, pages 43–8, for a more in-depth discussion on clinical audit. Link to Chapter 5, pages 59–64, for ideas and strategies on how to reflect and subsequently improve professional practice and patient care.

It is rare that paramedics are the only healthcare professionals involved in the patient's care; an interprofessional approach is the usual practice. It is necessary to disclose information to health and social care professionals when paramedic practitioners, for example, convey patients to accident and emergency (A&E) departments to provide the uninterrupted 'patient care pathway'. In such situations, a copy of the patient report form will be left in the department with the relevant A&E staff. Patients' consent in such situations should be sought, to enable disclosure of their information wherever possible. When patients are conveyed to hospital, their consent will have been obtained routinely in the vast majority of cases. It is accepted that by agreeing to be taken to hospital, disclosure of information relating to the patient will be shared by the ambulance clinician with those entitled to receive it.

There will be situations where the need for confidentiality has to be balanced against what is termed the 'public interest'. Under common law, practitioners are permitted to disclose personal information in order to support detection, investigation and punishment of serious crime and/or to prevent abuse or serious harm to others where they judge, on a case-by-case basis, that disclosure outweighs the obligation of confidentiality. Practitioners should consider each case on its own merits. On occasions, due to the nature of the incident, it may be difficult to make a decision. In such situations it may be necessary to seek legal or specialist advice from professional, regulatory or employing authorities' legal departments, who will seek further legal advice as required.

The NHS policy relating to confidentiality is grounded in guidance from Department of Health documents such as *Confidentiality: NHS Code of Practice* (DoH 2003a), *Guidance for Access to Health Records Requests* (DoH 2003b) and from the Information Commissioner: *Use and Disclosure of Health Data* (Information Commissions Office 2002).

Accountability

The Health Professions Order (DoH 2001: Part V, 21. 1a) states that we must 'establish and keep under review the standards of conduct, performance and ethics expected of registrants and prospective registrants and give them guidance on these matters as (we) see fit'. Every paramedic agreeing to go on the register has to confirm that they have read and agree to adhere to the standard explained in the standards of conduct, performance and ethics required by the Health Professions Council (2003). The areas covered within this document are outlined in Box 2.2.

Health Profession Council practice committees

The areas mentioned in Box 2.2 form the basis on which paramedics will be held accountable, should a complaint be made against them. The HPC has practice committees who look into allegations made against registered paramedics. There are three practice committees:

- First, the **investigating committee** normally looks at every allegation to decide whether there is a case to answer. If a case to answer is apparent, this committee

---

Box 2.2 A summary of the role of paramedics

Paramedics must:

- Protect the health and well being of people who use or need their services. Maintain high standards of conduct
- Always act in the best interests of their patients, users and clients. Respect the confidentiality of their patients, users and clients and maintain high standards of personal conduct. Provide any important information about conduct, competence and health
- Maintain a high level of performance. Keep their professional knowledge and skills up to date. Act within the limits of that knowledge and skills
- Maintain effective and proper communications with patients, clients and users and other healthcare professionals
- Effectively supervise tasks they have asked others to carry out. Get informed consent to treatment as required
- Keep accurate patient, client and user records. Deal fairly and safely with the risks of infection
- Limit their work or if necessary stop practising if they deem their performance or judgement is affected by health
- Maintain a high standard of ethics. They should endeavour to carry out their duties in a professional and ethical manner and behave with integrity and honesty.

(Adapted from HPC 2003)

---

deals with the case or decides to pass it onto one of the other two committees. It is expected that the investigating committee will always deal with cases of fraudulent or incorrect registration.

- Second, the **conduct and competence committee** normally deals with cases of misconduct and/or competence. They will also deal with matters arising from police cautions or criminal convictions.
- The third committee is known as **the health committee** and deals with cases of ill health.

The council, after dealing with each case, has the power to take action against a health professional if a case is established. Such action may involve removing the paramedic from the HPC register. Other action may include suspension from the register or restricting the individual's work or publicly cautioning him or her. Those prospective paramedics who are trying to join the register will not incur any penalties from the HPC during education, but will be unable to register if they do not reach the requirements of the HPC relating to the standards of conduct, performance and ethics that they have to reach in order to apply to be registered with the HPC. The standards will form part of their educational programme and may be assessed in theory and in the practice environment, depending on the structure and content of the programme validated by the HPC.

Consent

The *UK Ambulance Service Clinical Practice Guidelines* (JRCALC 2006) explain that patients have fundamental legal and ethical rights in determining what happens to their own bodies. Thus, the paramedic practitioner has to obtain valid consent in the majority of healthcare encounters.

Adult consent

For consent to be valid, a patient has to have the appropriate information and must be able to comprehend the procedure, treatment, intervention and so forth that is proposed by the paramedic practitioner. This means that the patient must be able to understand not only the procedure or treatment to be carried out, but also the consequences of such actions. This will allow the individual to consider the 'pros' and 'cons' of such situations and provide what is termed 'informed consent'.

Capacity

The comprehension required for informed consent is based around the patient's 'capacity' to understand the procedure being explained to him or her. The paramedic must have an understanding of the Mental Capacity Act (2005). This legislation will guide practice; paramedics need to read and understand the more succinct *Code of Practice* to the Act (Lord Chancellor 2007). If this proves difficult and there are still unanswered questions, the practitioner should seriously consider approaching his or her employer to facilitate workshops to explain the Act in more detail, as it is extremely crucial to practice competence and working within the law. Whilst the following quote is specifically concerned with people who have harmed themselves, the principle for education and training remains the same. Point 1.1.3.1 of the guidance published by the National Institute of Clinical Excellence (NICE) (2004) states, 'All healthcare professionals who have contact, in the emergency situation, with people who have self-harmed should be adequately trained to assess mental capacity and to make decisions about when treatment and care can be given without consent.' Ambulance clinicians may find NICE's guidance useful to know when trying to access training/continuing professional development on such complex, yet highly relevant issues.

The Mental Capacity Act (The Stationery Office 2005) confirms in legislation that it should be assumed that adults (aged 16 or over) have full legal capacity to make decisions for themselves (the right to autonomy) unless it can be shown that they lack capacity to make a decision for themselves at the time it needs to be made. The Code of Practice to the Act (Lord Chancellor 2007: 36) states that assessing capacity occurs in two stages:

Stage 1 Does the person have an impairment of, or a disturbance in the functioning of their brain or mind? e.g. concussion following head injury.

Stage 2 Does the impairment or disturbance mean that the person is unable to make a specific decision when they need to?

In answer to the question in Stage 2, the Act states that a person is unable to make a decision if they cannot:

- understand information about the decision made (the Act calls this 'relevant' information);
- retain that information in their mind;
- use or weigh that information as part of the decision-making process; or
- communicate their decision (by talking, using sign language or other means).

In circumstances described above, the Act (The Stationery Office 2005) provides a legal framework for how to act and make decisions on behalf of people who lack capacity to make specific decisions for themselves. In order to assess whether the patient understands the information given by the paramedic, the professional should explore the individual's ability to decipher what information is relevant in relation to the nature of the decision, to understand why the information is needed and the likely effects of deciding one way or another or making no decision at all. The Code of Practice to the Act (Lord Chancellor 2007) advises the practitioner to take time to enable the person to take in the information given to them. It also states that the practitioner must give an appropriate amount of information to the patient and must provide information relating to the risks of any treatment or non-treatment. With respect to 'taking time' with the patient, the Code does provide guidance on emergency situations. Code of Practice to the Act (Lord Chancellor 2007: 36) states:

> In emergency medical situations, urgent decisions will have to be made and immediate action taken in the person's best interests. In these situations, it may not be practical or appropriate to delay the treatment while trying to help the person make their own decisions. However, even in emergency situations, healthcare staff should try to communicate with the person and keep them informed of what is happening.

In light of the Mental Capacity Act (2005), JRCALC will be publishing some interim guidelines to assist clinicians with assessment and decision making.

The Act (2005) also introduces several new roles, bodies and powers, all supporting the Act. These include:

- Attorneys appointed under Lasting Power of Attorney (LPA). These individuals carry a great deal of power and, with respect to health care, have the responsibility to apply certain standards of care and skill (duty of care) when making decisions, respect confidentiality and carry out the donor's instructions, amongst many other responsibilities.
- The new Court of Protection, and court-appointed deputies. The paramedic may need to know when and how to make an application to the Court and certainly should have an understanding of the powers of the Court of Protection.
- Independent Mental Capacity Advocates (IMCA). This service is independent and is for people who lack capacity to make certain important decisions and, at the time such decisions need to be made, have no one else (other than paid staff) to support or represent them or to be consulted.

The paramedic, in the course of a lifetime career, is likely to meet many difficult and complex situations, so should have an understanding of the above powers or bodies. It is strongly recommended that any ambulance clinician in difficult circumstances and having problems with the issue of capacity should ask for advice from their ambulance NHS Trust or employer through the normal emergency channels within their service.

The Department of Health (2001) advises that consent must be given voluntarily without duress or undue influence from health professionals, relatives or friends. In order for the patient to give consent it does not have to be written, as this does not exclusively prove the consent is valid. Written evidence is used to record the patient's decision and the events which may have taken place.

Child consent

The Department of Health (2001) explains that before examining, treating or caring for a child the paramedic must seek consent. Young people aged 16 and 17 are presumed to have the competence to give consent for themselves. Younger children who understand fully what is involved in the proposed procedure can also give consent, although it is better if their parents are involved in the decision at the time it is being made. In other cases, someone with parental responsibility must give consent on the child's behalf, unless they cannot be reached in an emergency. If a 'competent child' consents to treatment, a parent cannot override that consent. Legally, a parent can consent if a competent child refuses, but it is likely that taking such a serious step will be rare. If you are unsure, obtain legal advice from your NHS Trust or employer, as consent concerning children can be very complex.

Patient refusal

Competent adult patients may refuse treatment (DoH 2001). The only exception to this rule is where treatment is for a mental disorder/illness and the patient is detained under the Mental Health Acts (DoH 1983, 2007). If a patient is not competent, then a paramedic may treat the patient if it is in her best interests. This may include the wishes of the patient when she was competent. People close to the patient may be able to give more information and help the practitioner make a balanced, well-informed decision in such circumstances.

Link to Chapter 3 for the theory and value of communication in patient and colleague encounters. Link to Chapter 8 where common conditions are explained, signs and symptoms explored, which will be useful for the paramedic to establish competence. The Mental Health Acts of 1983 and 2007 are discussed in more detail and useful web addresses provided.

Conclusion

It is accepted that the role of modern paramedics brings with it a number of important legal areas within their scope of practice. Paramedics need to be aware of the consequences of their actions and be able to maintain a professional, legal and ethical approach at all times. Understanding the law is particularly important as the broadening of paramedic skills continues to develop. The HPC seeks to provide a framework within which paramedics are able to practise to the highest standards and simultaneously maintain their accountability to patients, clients and other professionals. This chapter represents an overview of some of the most common legal and ethical dilemmas facing the paramedic in the twenty-first century. Many of the areas require further investigation and wider reading, in order to obtain a more comprehensive understanding of the issues covered in this chapter.

Chapter key points

- Ethical dilemmas are part of everyday practice within the NHS.
- There are differences between paramedic guidance and that of other healthcare professionals.
- Paramedic ethical dilemmas occur across the lifespan, due to the nature of the role.
- Paramedics require a good understanding of their ethical responsibilities in relation to the role, in order to practise in a safe, competent and professional manner.

References and suggested reading

DoH (Department of Health) (1983) *Mental Health Act.* London: Department of Health.

DoH (2001) *Consent: What You Have a Right to Expect. A Guide for Adults.* London: Department of Health.

DoH (2001) *The Health Professions Order.* London: Department of Health.

DoH (2003a) *Confidentiality: National Health Service Code of Practice.* London: Department of Health.

DoH (2003b) *Guidance for Access to Health Records Requests under the Data Protection Act 1998,* Version 2. London: Department of Health.

DoH (2007) *Mental Health Act.* London: Department of Health.

Health Professions Council (2003) *Standards of Conduct, Performance and Ethics. Your Duties as a Registrant.* London: Health Professions Council.

JRCALC (Joint Royal Colleges Ambulance Liaison Committee) (2006) *United Kingdom Ambulance Service Clinical Practice Guidelines.* London: Joint Royal Colleges Ambulance Liaison Committee/ The Ambulance Service Association (ASA).

Her Majesty's Stationery Office (1998) *Data Protection Act.* London: HMSO.

Information Commissions Office (2002) *Use and Disclosure of Health Data. Guidance on the Application of the Data Protection Act 1998.* London: HMSO.

Lord Chancellor (2007) *Mental Capacity Act 2005 Code of Practice.* Issued by the Lord Chancellor on 23 April 2007 in accordance with sections 42 and 43 of the Act. London: The Stationery Office.

National Institute for Clinical Excellence (2004) *Self Harm. The Short-term Physical and Psychological Management and Secondary Prevention of Self-harm in Primary and Secondary Care.* Clinical Guideline 16. London: NICE.

The Stationery Office (2005) *The Mental Capacity Act.* London: The Stationery Office.

3

Interpersonal communication: a foundation of practice
Paul Street

Topics covered:

- Introduction
- Why is this relevant?
- Basic model of interpersonal communication
- Verbal communication
- Non-verbal communication
- An advanced model of interpersonal communication
- Conclusion
- Chapter key points
- References and suggested reading

Introduction

Why is communication important? Communication is important because it is such an integral part of our lives it is impossible to think of any situation when an individual does not communicate in some way (Hartley 1999; Ellis 2003). Without interpersonal communication ambulance clinicians would not be able to talk to patients, know the location of their next call, or hand over a patient to the staff in an accident and emergency department.

Why is this relevant?

The ability to communicate, therefore, is seen as an essential skill required by ambulance clinicians, nurses and all healthcare practitioners (Ellis 2003; Health Professions Council 2003, 2007; Benner 2006; Bickley and Szilagyi 2007). Despite communication being such a fundamental part of personal and professional practice, each year the National Health Service receives a large numbers of complaints from patients about poor communication (Department of Health 2007). It seems evident, then, that health practitioners need to be constantly aware of not only what they say, but how they say it, so placing communication in the forefront of practice.

Definition of communication

Communication has multiple meanings, all of which emphasize different things; take any one and it may limit your appreciation of the subject (Hartley 1999). For example, communication is the transfer of information from one person to another.

 Stop and think – How might you communicate information to one of your friends? How does your example 'fit' with the definition above?

Basic model of interpersonal communication

The most rudimentary model of interpersonal communication proposes that a sender sends a message that is received by a receiver (Ellis 2003). The sender will formulate a message and send it to the receiver using verbal and non-verbal means of communication (see Figure 3.1).

Sender ⟶ Message ⟶ Receiver
(Person A)   (Person B)

Figure 3.1 Model of communication

The message is the information being sent from the sender to the receiver. It can be anything from an emotion to a formal instruction. The verbal message, in many cases, is not thought out in full prior to it being communicated. If you think of how you speak to your friends and colleagues, do you formulate all of what you want to say, then say it, or are you able apparently just to think and talk simultaneously as the conversation progresses? Much of our communication may appear, therefore, to be spontaneous and not scripted and seems to be in response to the context in which communication occurs. Direct messages are the clearest and easiest ones for the receiver to understand, because they are unambiguous and based on a common language between the sender and receiver. Multiple messages, however, are often complex, with a combination of verbal and non-verbal meanings being sent (Ellis 2003). Receivers uses their senses (hearing, sight and touch, etc.) to receive the message, which they then need to interpret. Hence if the receiver, or indeed the sender, has reduced levels of these senses then alterations in the way the message is sent may be required to compensate for this (Benner 2006).

Verbal communication

Verbal communication is, in essence, a deliberate conscious process because people select the words from their vocabulary that they want to use in order to communicate. This is clearly evident in Bernstein's (1971) seminal work, which established that people from different social classes have different language codes made up of vocabulary and speech patterns. This work suggested that people of higher social classes have an elaborate language code and complex vocabulary, while those in lower social classes have a more restricted language code with a more limited vocabulary. This has implications for both the sender and the receiver in terms of how they send and interpret the message because of the language code and vocabulary they possess. Further, the context in which communication occurs may also influence the vocabulary and language used in it, because of the social and professional expectations placed on clinicians (Limmer *et al.* 2005; Bledsoe *et al.* 2007). Hence, ambulance clinicians are required to use professional-level vocabulary with colleagues, yet be able to translate that to meet the needs of patients and relatives who may have various levels of understanding of that terminology, different levels of cognitive development and varied communication abilities.

Link to Chapter 11 to read more about the factors affecting people's social development.

Verbal features of communication

The meaning of the messages we communicate may change depending on the paralinguistic features used to convey them (Ellis 2003). The paralinguistic features outlined in Figure 3.2 are used to emphasize the meaning of the message the sender wishes to place on it.

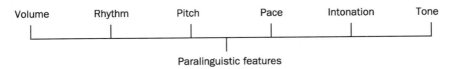

Figure 3.2 Paralinguistic features of communication

Evidently, when the sender speaks to send a verbal message it needs to be sent at a volume at which the receiver can hear it. The volume used to send a message may vary depending on the situation, for example two ambulance clinicians talking at a busy roadside would need a louder volume than those talking to a patient in his home. Further ensuring an appropriate volume level is important in terms of the effectiveness of the communication: too loud and a patient may think you are shouting at them, too soft and they may not hear you at all. Both of these could limit the patient's ability to interpret the correct meaning of the message, let alone having the potential to leave the patient with a lasting negative impression of how health practitioners communicate.

Closely linked to volume is pitch; usually the louder the volume the higher the pitch of voice. If these two elements are then linked to a fast pace of speaking they could then, paralinguistically, communicate a sense of urgency (Hartley 1999), but if taken further they could communicate a sense of stress or panic. Thus, possible consequences of health practitioners using a raised volume, pitch and pace are that the people receiving the message may potentially think the situation is serious, or perhaps that practitioners may be unsure of what they are doing. These changes may be, in part, due to alterations in the practitioner's stress levels during any patient interaction, particularly if it is a stressful one; moreover, the more the practitioner feels under pressure the more these features may appear in the voice. Hence, controlling the voice by having a calm paced rhythm and tone in the voice at an appropriate volume may then communicate confidence (Mistovich *et al.* 2000).

Changing the meaning of a verbal message

So as paralinguistic features can change the meaning of the spoken message unintentionally, they can equally be used to change it intentionally. For example, the meaning of the statement 'I'll see you outside the library at eight' can be changed from a question to a command by altering the emphasis in the voice; likewise, by changing the tone and emphasis the following statement could be praising or insulting a student: 'He's an excellent student'. So here the words of an appropriate message may be spoken, but the emphasis and paralinguistic features may give an alternative meaning to that message. Hence, all health practitioners need to consider which words they use and how they emphasize them to give clear, caring, empathetic and assertive messages to patients and not ones that indicate the clinician's frustrations, attitudes or assumptions.

Link to Chapter 6 for information on the use of reflection within the role of ambulance clinician. Consider the importance of reflecting on the paralinguistics during certain types of calls.

 Stop and think – Which paralinguistic features do you use when you communicate the following things:

- To arrange a time and date to meet a friend for a drink.
- To suggest you don't believe a friend's story, without saying 'I don't believe you.'
- To give an instruction to a colleague, to give a piece of equipment to you.
- Would your friend or colleagues say the same things about you or not?

Non-verbal communication

Communication does not only occur verbally; people instinctively communicate non-verbally when they are talking (Argyle 1988). Non-verbal communication, in a similar way to the paralinguistic features of verbal communication, can replace, supplement or contradict the meaning of the verbal message being sent (Ellis 2003). Many non-verbal cues are unconscious manifestations of thoughts and feelings. Consequently, it is difficult for individuals to have total conscious control over their non-verbal cues and to some degree they will always communicate non-verbal messages they are unaware of, even if they are acutely aware of their own body language (Hartley 1999). Thrower (2002) talks of this in terms of everybody having a blind and unconscious 'self', in which individuals are unaware of elements of their behaviour and only gain insight into this when someone else brings it to their attention. Thus, feedback from colleagues is a useful way of becoming more aware of your communication skills and appreciating how you are seen by others.

It is possible for two ambulance clinicians to communicate with each other exclusively through non-verbal means, with a smile, a wave or a gesture, for example. But it would be more difficult for these two people in the same context to communicate only through vocal means. This is primarily because our physical gestures and non-verbal cues are unconsciously linked to our verbal expression (Bledsoe *et al.* 2007). At some level, verbal communication can appear to be isolated when using the telephone. But if you watch someone talking on the phone they don't just talk; they also use their hands, gestures and facial expressions too. Of course, these non-verbal cues are not usually observable by the person on the other end of the phone. It is evident that the sender is still using a mix of verbal and non-verbal cues; it is just that the receiver cannot see them. This supports the assertion that all interpersonal communication is an amalgam of verbal and non-verbal cues acting as carriers for the message (Ellis 2003).

Eye contact

Eye contact is one form of non-verbal communication (Argyle 1988). It is an important way in which people initiate and maintain communication and its use by ambulance clinicians can show they are interested in their patients (Limmer *et al.* 2005). Usually the receiver will maintain eye contact with the sender for the main part of the message, while the sender will have periods when she looks away and returns to have eye contact with the receiver (Ellis 2003). Consequently, if someone is not looking at you when you are speaking it may be a sign that they are not listening. Although, if they are avoiding eye contact, but demonstrating they are listening by giving suitable verbal responses with appropriate paralinguistic features, it may be that in this situation it may be culturally insensitive or even rude to maintain eye contact (Limmer *et al.* 2005). Another complication of eye contact is that it can have different meanings depending on the context in which it is used. Direct prolonged eye contact by both people involved can be a sign of aggression or alternatively a sign of attraction. This illustrates the fact that any single element of non-verbal communication has to be considered in relation to the other non-verbal and verbal cues exhibited in that situation in order to interpret the message correctly.

Facial expression

In conjunction with eye contact, the face is one of the most expressive parts of a human body and feelings are often clearly communicated through the face alone; for example anger, joy and surprise are quite often easy to identify non-verbally through facial expressions. It is evident that ambulance clinicians will be faced with situations that they find shocking, fearful or surprising and there is a strong likelihood that they may display those emotions through their facial expressions. It is noticeable that patients can recognize the emotions and mood states displayed by the clinicians caring for them (Bickley and Szilagyi 2007). Again the implications are that health practitioners need to have the self-awareness to understand the non-verbal cues they may exhibit.

Link to Chapter 6 Consider the importance of reflecting on the reactions that patients and family members have demonstrated or expressed as a result of your facial expressions during certain types of calls. Have you observed a colleague make unprofessional and inappropriate facial expressions, how did this make you feel? How might you 'tackle' this, if it happened again?

Gestures and posture

Alongside facial expressions both gestures and posture can emphasize and clarify the meaning of the spoken message (Hartley 1999). People often use their hands to gesture when they are speaking, waving as they say goodbye, for example. Some gestures like pointing can be problematic depending on the context in which they have been used; pointing to a piece of equipment can be appropriate but pointing at a patient may not be. Equally, using large gestures may convey enthusiasm, but used extensively in a patient interaction can move the focus of the situation away from the patient to the ambulance clinician, which may or may not be helpful in some situations.

Posture includes the way you stand, sit and position your body (Argyle 1988). It has particular relevance when you as a clinician adopt a posture or position in relation to a patient. It is generally accepted that, if possible, when talking to patients you should have an open posture, i.e. without your arms or legs crossed, as an open posture suggests you are willing to communicate with the other person, as would positioning yourself at the same level as the patient in order to maintain eye contact on an equal level (Limmer et al. 2005; Bledsoe et al. 2007). Nevertheless, using this posture may not always be particularly appropriate at the scene of a road traffic accident, but the principles can be applied to many other situations in which ambulance clinicians communicate with patients and relatives.

The position or angle of the head can also communicate meaning (Hartley 1999). Tilting the head forward combined with looking over the top of a pair of glasses can be seen as intimidating, while inclining the head to one side slightly can be perceived as a sign of interest. Both posture and gestures can have a positive effect on establishing and maintaining good communication, especially if used in combination with eye contact. If these are used appropriately they can suggest you are concerned for the patient and are willing to listen to him, but if used unwisely they can also alienate a patient or relative, because they can suggest you could be uncaring and unwilling to listen.

Personal space and touch

People also can communicate by how closely they stand or sit next to another person. This is referred to as personal space or proximity (Argyle 1988). Generally during social interaction people who do not know each other tend to stand approximately at an arm's length away from each other (Ellis 2003). This distance is often reduced when the people know each other, or when one person gives permission directly or indirectly for someone to invade their personal space and touch them. Being too close can cause discomfort and unease and be perceived as threatening, even if touch is not involved.

Additionally, touch is another significant element of non-verbal communication for ambulance clinicians (Bledsoe *et al.* 2007), because much of the care given requires touch: placing a blood pressure cuff, stabilizing a C-spine, for example. This procedural touch is often easier for the clinician and the patient, providing explanations and consent are obtained. Although touch is an instinctive form of communication, it can be misinterpreted and become problematic, so be sure to touch patients in socially acceptable parts of the body (the hands, for example, if that is clinically appropriate), until you have direct or implied consent to touch them elsewhere (Mistovitch *et al.* 2000).

Link to Chapter 2 for more detailed explanation of the concept of consent and the paramedic's role.

 Stop and think Thinking about these non-verbal cues, how else might you be able to identify the following:

- someone was not listening to you;
- a colleague was interested in what you were saying;
- the person you were talking to was worried;
- a colleague tells you to do something quickly?

Link to Chapter 6 Consider your posture, use of touch, proximity and angle of your head in relation to different pre-hospital calls. Can you improve your communication skills?

An advanced model of interpersonal communication

In light of the issues of verbal and non-verbal communication the message–sender–receiver model appears to be simplistic, as the nature of communication is far from being this straightforward. Furthermore, interpersonal communication is rarely one way, because the sender will not only send a message, but also receive the response message from the receiver. Interpersonal communication, therefore, is a continuous cycle of sending and receiving messages, with the sender also being a receiver and vice versa (Hartley 1999), as seen in Figure 3.3.

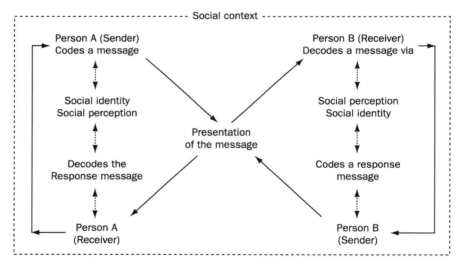

Figure 3.3 Model of interpersonal communication
Source: Adapted from Hartley (1999)

Hartley's (1999) model suggests that communication does not occur in a vacuum; it always takes place in a 'social context' that will influence both the sender and receiver, and therefore how the message is formulated, sent and received. For example, when you have a conversation with a colleague in the context of an ambulance station coffee room about a clinical incident, you may be talking freely in a relaxed way. But when being interviewed in the same ambulance station by a Station Officer in her office about the same incident, the change in context may increase the degree of formality and so you may use more formal verbal and non-verbal communication.

In addition, the model demonstrates that the communication process is complicated by the fact that the sender will encode the message they send through the words, speech patterns and body language they use to send it and give the message the required meaning (Hartley 1999). The receiver then has to decode those elements to understand the message he has been sent. It is here that the receiver may misinterpret the message and send an inappropriate response back to the sender, particularly if the initial message contained mixed messages within it. Adding to the complexity of communication further, the processes of encoding and decoding messages are influenced by many factors within our social identity, personality, values, beliefs, gender, culture, status, to name just a few (Hartley 1999). These arise out of the person's primary, secondary and professional socialization and will result in people conforming to the expected role and behaviours of any particular social or professional role (Gabe *et al.* 2004; Bickley and Szilagyi 2007).

Link to Chapter 11 for further reading on the process of socialization.

Furthermore, how individuals perceive themselves and the context they are in can also influence the way they encode and decode messages, which is further compounded by the way they perceive themselves within that particular situation at that particular time. These factors all influence how you encode and decode messages. Hence Hartley's (1999) model represents a more comprehensive model of interpersonal communication and helps provide a way of viewing how socialization, social identify and the communication context will affect the way a message is encoded, transmitted, decoded and interpreted.

 Stop and think Think back to the first definition. What does interpersonal communication mean to you now?

Conclusion

Interpersonal communication is a complex exchange of information between people who constantly send and receive messages to and from each other. Interpersonal communication consists of verbal and non-verbal elements. Both the verbal and non-verbal elements of the message can be altered by the use of paralinguistic features and non-verbal cues. It is important to remember, therefore, that verbal and non-verbal communication are inextricably linked and it is the way a person uses them in combination that impacts on their interactions with their patients and colleagues. It is this combination that allows ambulance clinicians to communicate a range of messages effectively from the very subtle to the blatantly obvious. But what is important is that the communication is effective and sensitive to the situation and the people involved within it. It seems evident, then, that health practitioners need to be constantly aware not only of what they say, but how they say it, so placing communication in the forefront of practice.

Chapter key points

- We are always in a state of communicating something to someone.
- Communication is a mix of verbal and non-verbal elements; these act as carriers of the messages we send and receive.
- The way we formulate, send, receive and interpret messages is influenced by our values, beliefs, social identity, perceptions and the context in which the communication occurs.
- Communication is a fundamental and vital part of all healthcare practitioners' practice, because care and treatment cannot effectively occur without communication of some kind.

References and suggested reading

Argyle, M. (1988) *Bodily Communication*, 2nd edn. London: Routledge.

Benner, R.W. (2006) Communications and documentation, in B.E. Bledsoe and R.W. Benner (eds) *Critical Care Ambulance Clinician*. New Jersey, NJ: Prentice-Hall.

Bernstein, B. (1971) *Class, Codes and Control, Volume 1*. London: Routledge & Kegan Paul.

Bickley, L.S. and Szilagyi, P.G. (2007) Interviewing and health history, in L.S. Bickley, and P.G. Szilagyi, (eds) *Bates' Guide to Physical Examination and History Taking*. Philadelphia, PA: Lippincott Williams & Wilkins.

Bledsoe, B.E., Porter, R.S. and Cherry, R.A. (2007) *Essentials of Ambulance Clinician Care*, 2nd edn. New Jersey, NJ Prentice-Hall.

DoH (Department of Health) (2007) *Hospital Activity Statistics 2003–04*. http://www.performance.doh.gov.uk/hospitalactivity/data_requests/nhs_complaints.html (Accessed 17 June 2007).

Ellis, R. (2003) Defining communication, in R. Ellis, B. Gates and N. Kenworthy (eds) *Interpersonal Communication in Nursing: Theory and Practice*, 2nd edn. Edinburgh: Churchill Livingstone.

Gabe, J., Bury, M. and Elston, M. (2004) *Key Concepts in Medical Sociology*. London: Sage Publications.

Hartley, P. (1999) *Interpersonal Communication*, 2nd edn. London: Routledge.

Health Professions Council (2003) *Standards of Conduct, Performance and Ethics*. London: HPC.

Health Professions Council (2007) *Standards of Proficiency for Paramedics*. London: HPC.

Limmer, D., O'Keefe, F. and Dickinson, E. (2005) Communications, in D. Limmer, M.F. O'Keefe and E. Dickinson (eds) *Emergency Care*, 10th edn. New Jersey, NJ: Prentice-Hall.

Mistovich, J.J., Hafen, B.Q. and Karren, K.S. (2000) Communication, in J.J. Mistovich, B.Q. Hafen and K.S. Karren (eds) *Pre-hospital Emergency Care*. New Jersey, NJ: Prentice-Hall.

Thrower, C. (2002) Understanding ourselves, in R. Hodston and P.M. Simpson (2002) *Foundations of Nursing Practice: Making a Difference*. Basingstoke: Palgrave Macmillan.

4

Professional issues affecting practice
Rachael Donohoe and Amanda Blaber

Topics covered:

- Introduction
- Why is this relevant?
- Anti-discriminatory practice
- Clinical governance
- Clinical audit
- Evidence-based practice
- Conclusion
- Chapter key points
- References, suggested reading and useful websites

Introduction

This chapter is a mix of issues that affect the way you practise in the pre-hospital environment. Some of the areas, like clinical audit, will have a direct effect and you will be involved with it on a daily basis. Others, such as anti-discriminatory practice and evidence-based practice, are implicit in the way that you conduct yourself, how you relate to others and the quality of the care that you provide. The inclusion of these issues clearly reflects the *professional* nature of paramedic practice. These professional issues will be addressed in higher education diplomate/graduate programmes of study. Student paramedics need an understanding of these issues and an appreciation of their importance, in order to implement the principles within their everyday conduct and practice.

Why is this relevant?

Everything the ambulance clinician does in practice is subject to the rigours of clinical audit. It is important that all healthcare practitioners are aware of what happens to their documentation and how this influences future recommendations. The discussion of anti-discriminatory practice should be at the forefront of clinicians' minds on a daily basis. It is worthwhile to review your practice, raise self-awareness and challenge views in order to improve the patient experience. Evidence-based practice is critical to the role of the ambulance clinician – indeed, any healthcare professional. Evidence-based practice influences protocols, policy development and treatment for patients. Striving to obtain an appreciation of evidence-based practice theory will assist the clinician to understand the role of evidence-based practice within twenty-first-century health care. This chapter aims to raise your awareness of these issues, help you to understand the importance of the issues to pre-hospital care, invite you to question your own behaviour and leave you wanting to explore the areas in more detail for yourselves.

Anti-discriminatory practice

Definition of anti-discriminatory practice

An approach to practice which seeks to reduce, undermine or eliminate discrimination and oppression, specifically in terms of challenging sexism, racism, ageism and disabilism and other forms of discrimination encountered in practice (Thompson 2006: 40).

Definition of stereotype

Comes from the Greek stereo meaning solid. Tupos means type, oversimplified, biased. The word has its origins in the printing trade for a solid metallic plate which was difficult to alter once cast (Oxford 2006).

Anti-discriminatory practice is a term used in health care but what does it mean both legally and professionally to pre-hospital care personnel? Any healthcare professional has the ethical, legal, moral and professional responsibilities to deal with all patients/clients in a way that does not discriminate against them, as described in paramedic standard of proficiency 1a.2 (HPC 2007). How can you as clinicians be sure that you are acting in an anti-discriminatory manner? The next few pages will provide some definitions and aim to broaden your thinking about the ways in which a person can feel discriminated against.

The definition by Thompson (2006) clearly identifies areas of daily life and societal structure that make us individuals. These areas are represented visually in Figure 4.1. All of us can identify areas where we differ from our friends, family and colleagues. These differences can form the basis of social division, if we are subject to discrimination because of our membership to one or more areas mentioned in Figure 4.1.

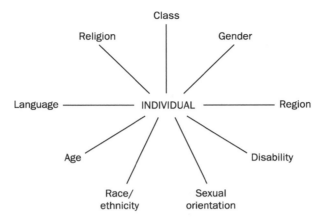

Figure 4.1 Areas of our lives where we may be subjected to discrimination

 Stop and think – Consider yourself in relation to Figure 4.1. Can you identify any areas of your life where you feel you are discriminated against? Explore how this makes you feel.

Processes of discrimination

Stereotyping

Broad categories are used to identify or classify people or objects on an everyday basis. This process can be called typification. Categorizing people/objects often makes it easier for us to make sense of our society. For example, if asked about disability, people may identify a 'typical' disabled person as being a wheelchair user: this is far from the case, as there are many other forms of disability. The typifications created can become very fixed and rigid; when this occurs stereotypes are created. When these stereotypes are accepted by us and are used on a daily basis, we tend not to discover the information needed to treat the person as an individual, as we tend not to question what we think we know. This obviously affects the level of individualized care that an ambulance clinician can achieve, even in the relatively short amount of time that is spent with each patient/client.

 Stop and think – about the stereotypes you assume on a daily basis. Do you think you have challenged your assumptions to discover the 'real' individual?

Once established, stereotypes are resistant to change, are often negative and have the potential to be oppressive. Perhaps the biggest danger is that we often do not notice stereotypes being used by ourselves and others. These will affect our perceptions and actions on a daily basis and require questioning.

Marginalization

Groups of people that feel oppressed, excluded from decision making and lacking power can be described as being marginalized from mainstream society. For example, people with disabilities may feel marginalized from society because of the social attitudes that devalue people with disabilities. Due to inconsiderate design/finances, people with disabilities are often prevented from accessing certain buildings and transport networks. This demonstrates the lack of societal willingness to enable people with disabilities to participate fully in social, political and economic areas of life.

Invisibilization

This refers to the language and imagery used to represent certain groups. We are constantly bombarded by media images of powerful dominant groups who are associated with positions of power, status, influence and prestige, such as politicians and world leaders. Other groups of people, for example older people and people with disabilities, are rarely represented in this light. Without being challenged, the dominant groups will continue to define and dominate society.

Infantilization

Power, rights, resources and life chances are allocated in accordance with our age. Imposing a child-like status to an adult can be seen as a form of disempowerment, a denial of citizenship and rights. This is especially important when considering your communication skills when caring for people with a learning disability or older members of society. Examples of this are phrases like 'Can you tell me where he is in pain?' (asking the carer rather than the patient), or 'He's a lovely old boy.' Such comments made by healthcare professionals may not be intended to be discriminatory, but do reinforce stereotypes. It is intended that practitioners should review the language and terminology they use.

Medicalization

In the past, many people with a learning disability lived in long-stay hospitals where they were in the care of the medical profession and allied carers, reinforcing the position of power these so-called experts had over this group of people. The hospital also ascribes the status of 'ill' to those admitted; this has significant implications for them, where this is not necessarily the case. This medicalization results in a 'label' being applied to groups of people, which can reduce people's status in society.

Link to Chapter 12, pages 185–190, for a clearer explanation of these concepts

Stop and think – about people you have cared for. Have you ever come across or experienced some of the issues above?

Diversity

Definition of diversity

Thompson (2006: 41) defines diversity as a term 'being used to emphasize the differences between individuals and across groups and the fact that such differences are best seen as assets to be valued and affirmed, rather than as problems to be solved'.

Thompson (2006) sees diversity as an important discrimination issue and highlights the consequences that a lack of sensitivity to diversity can lead to:

- Alienating people – making some groups feel they do not belong in society.
- Invalidating people – creating the impression or feeling in some people that their perspective or experience is not valid because they differ from the mainstream.
- Missing key issues – because we are not sensitive to how important they are for the person or the group.
- Becoming part of the problem – failing to challenge discrimination and therefore playing a part in its continuance.

All NHS Trusts have policies on diversity and you may have the opportunity to undertake further education in this area. Make sure you are familiar with the policy of your local NHS Trust. In addition to reading, there are some things Thompson (2002) recommends that you think about and act upon in your daily work to affirm diversity and improve the individualized care that you give to patients:

- Be wary of stereotypes.
- Take steps to learn about other perspectives.
- Focus on dignity.
- Consider your own power.
- Review your practice.
- Ask for feedback.
- Work together.

Obviously this can be applied within workplaces and with the people who are your colleagues on a daily basis. Thompson (2003) considers that there are four key principles to valuing diversity within the workplace:

1   People work best when they feel valued.

2   People feel most valued when they believe that their individual and group differ-
     ences have been taken into account.

3   The ability to learn from people regarded as 'different' is the key to becoming
     fully empowered.

4   When people feel valued and empowered, they are able to build relationships in
     which they work together interdependently.

The legal framework

There are a number of Acts that are in place to support and protect people from
discrimination. It is wise for any person working with members of the public to be
aware of the content and main points of relevant Acts. The websites listed below often
provide a summary of the main points of each Act. The following list of Acts is by no
means 'all you need to know' but should serve as a starting point to your own investi-
gations and further enquiry:

Equal Pay Act 1970

> www.womenandequalityunit.gov.uk/legislation/equal_pay_act.html

Sex Discrimination Act 1975

> www.womenandequalityunit.gov.uk/legislation/discrimination_act.html

Race Relations Act 1976

> www.cre.gov/legal/rra.html

Disability Discrimination Act 1995

> www.opsi.gov.uk.acts/acts1995/1995050.html

Disability Rights Commission Act 1999

> www.opsi.gov.uk/acts/acts1999/19990017.html

Race Relations (Amendment Act) 2000

> www.opsi.gov.uk/acts/acts2000/20000034.html

Human Rights Act 1998

> www.opsi.gov.uk/acts/acts1998/19980042.html OR
> www.direct.gov.uk

The Employment Equality (Age) Regulations 2006

> www.dti.gov.uk

Anti-discriminatory practice should be implicit in the way ambulance clinicians work.
It is hoped that this section of the chapter has heightened your awareness of the
subject and encouraged you to examine your working practices. The remaining sections of this chapter are predominantly concerned with quality of practice. The first
subject to be discussed is clinical governance.

Clinical governance

Clinical governance is a framework for ensuring that quality is at the heart of the NHS. It is generally recognized that prior to its introduction in 1997, there was a distinct lack of organizational responsibility for quality within the NHS. The focal points for organizational managers were financial matters and performance targets (Donaldson and Gray 1998) and it has been argued that the NHS was managed as though clinical matters were peripheral (Oyebode *et al.* 1999a). That being said, there were some attempts to address quality during the early 1990s. For example, a responsibility was placed on doctors to participate in medical audit (Department of Health 1989) and through the 1991 Patient's Charter, patients' rights and guarantees of standards of care were introduced (Donaldson and Gray 1998).

When the new Labour government came to power in 1997, it began a major reform of the NHS. It published a White Paper: *The New NHS: Modern, Dependable* (Department of Health 1997: Ch.3, point 3.2), which sets out a ten-year modernization strategy that focuses on quality patient care and introduces the concept of clinical governance. This paper states that 'Every part of the NHS, and everyone who works in it, should take responsibility for working to improve quality. This must be quality in its broadest sense: doing the right things, at the right time, for the right people, and doing them right – first time.' The following year, the consultation document *A First Class Service: Quality in the NHS* (Department of Health 1998) outlines the vision for clinical governance. It describes how standards for quality care would be achieved through National Service Frameworks and the National Institute for clinical Excellence (NICE). In March 1999, the responsibilities of all NHS organizations under clinical governance were detailed in *Clinical Governance: Quality in the New NHS* (DoH 1999a).

The importance of quality was further reinforced by the Health Act of June 1999 (Section 18), which establishes a statutory duty of quality, requiring NHS Trusts to meet more than their financial statutory duties (DoH 1999b). Through the Act, NHS Trusts are obligated to put in place and maintain arrangements for monitoring and improving the standards of care they provide.

What is clinical governance?

Definition of clinical governance

A framework through which NHS organizations are accountable for continuously improving the quality of their services and safeguarding high standards of care by creating an environment in which excellence in clinical care will flourish (Department of Health 1998: Ch.3: 2).

Clinical governance is a mechanism that aims to improve standards of clinical practice and increase patient and public confidence in the NHS.

Clinical governance is not simply concerned with achieving and maintaining high standards, but with continuously improving them to create an environment of clinical excellence. It has been defined as 'a mission not just to do well, but to do better' (Donaldson 2000: 7).

The key principles of clinical governance are: clear lines of responsibility and accountability for the quality of clinical care; a comprehensive programme of quality improvement activities; clear policies for managing risks; and procedures for identifying and addressing poor performance. Clinical governance focuses on reducing variations in practice, providing equal access to services, and ensuring that clinical decisions are based on the most up-to-date evidence of what is clinically effective.

Clinical governance is of direct relevance to every NHS Trust and every member of staff concerned with providing patient care or support services. Clinical governance operates mainly at a local level and provides a structured, consistent approach to clinical quality management. As well as bringing together organizational, managerial and clinical processes, clinical governance involves integrating and enhancing a wide range of existing (previously separate) systems, such as clinical audit, complaints procedures and risk management, to improve patient care. Under clinical governance, NHS Trust Chief Executives hold ultimate accountability for the quality of services provided by their organizations. Each NHS Trust Board has a clinical governance sub-committee with a designated senior clinician responsible for ensuring and monitoring clinical governance systems. Clinical governance reports are provided to the Trust Board and these are treated as importantly as financial reports. Each Trust is also required to provide information on how it assures quality care as part of its annual report.

A National Audit Office report (2003) of the implementation of clinical governance in the NHS highlighted a number of positive outcomes. The report states that clinical governance has resulted in quality being viewed as a corporate concern; that there is greater accountability of clinicians and managers for clinical performance and quality issues, greater involvement of patients and staff in decision making, and a culture change towards more open and collaborative ways of working. Most importantly, the report demonstrates that clinical governance has resulted in improvements in clinical practice and patient care.

The key components of clinical governance

It is helpful to view clinical governance as an 'umbrella' beneath which there are a number of key components that combine to make a quality organization. The key components are often described in terms of 'seven pillars' – the supporting mechanisms that need to be in place and maintained by coherent processes, strategies and activities, for effective clinical governance to be achieved:

Clinical effectiveness
Clinical effectiveness is about ensuring that interventions and treatments are based on the most recent evidence of what constitutes 'best practice', as far as such evidence is available. This involves the effective implementation of evidence-based guidelines and using research and evaluation to inform and support changes in clinical practice. Clinical effectiveness represents a system in which clinical decisions, guidelines and health policies are no longer based on professional opinion alone.

Risk management

Risk management involves minimizing and controlling risks to the patient, the practitioner and the organization. In order to manage risks effectively, robust, systematic processes are used to monitor, quickly identify and deal with clinical risks and adverse incidents, including poor clinical performance and practice. Effective risk management incorporates an open environment in which staff are willing and able to report adverse events, as well as a complaints system that is accessible to all patients. In order to truly manage risks, it is necessary for an organization and its staff to reflect on their practices, learn from mistakes and take action to avoid recurrences.

Clinical audit

Clinical audit is the principal method by which clinical quality and quality improvement is measured. It involves reviewing clinical practice and making changes to practice where necessary. Clinical audit has been described as one of the cornerstones of clinical governance (Oyebode *et al.* 1999b) and is described in more detail in a later section of this chapter.

Patient and public involvement

As users, or potential users, of NHS services, patients and the public can provide important insights into the quality of care that is being provided, and can have valuable ideas and suggestions for improving services. Clinical governance requires NHS Trusts to consult and listen to patients and the public, and give them the opportunity to influence the way in which services are provided and developed.

Education and training

High-quality care depends on high-quality education and training. In the medical arena, new developments occur at such a fast pace that a large amount of what is taught becomes quickly outdated. Continuing professional development is essential in keeping staff up to date with new developments, treatments and interventions, and enables them to perform their role effectively. Important aspects of continuing professional development include: a commitment by the organization and its staff to professional development; a high level of organizational support for staff in their development; and an environment in which staff are encouraged to be constructively self-critical and to identify their own development needs.

Link to Chapter 5 for strategies to help the student reflect on issues. Link to Chapter 16 for other aspects of continuing professional development.

Information management

The NHS has access to a vast amount of information about patients, medical conditions, treatments and interventions. Robust and accurate clinical data are essential for a number of purposes including research, monitoring and assessing performance and quality, and informing decision making. Effective information management ensures that such data are generated, collected and reported in a systematic way, and that information is available for use by clinicians, managers, service users and the public. Information management also encompasses the effective communication and dissemination of information between health professionals and managers, both within and across NHS organizations. This enables consistency in care and the sharing of best practice, ideas and innovations.

> Link to Chapter 3 for communication theory.

Staffing and staff management

A high-quality organization needs to be staffed by high-quality people. Effective staffing and staff management involves a number of things including: good recruitment and induction processes; systems for managing, developing and motivating staff; good working environments; and robust human resources policies to protect both the individual and the organization. It should also incorporate an organizational culture in which staff are listened to and valued.

> **Stop and think** – Consider the 'seven pillars' above. Are they all reflected within the structure of your NHS Trust?

Governance monitoring

The process of external, independent review is a valuable way of providing assurances to NHS organizations, their patients and the public that services are being monitored and are of a high standard. The Commission for Health Improvement (CHI) was established through the 1999 Health Act to provide such assurances. CHI was an independent body whose remit included conducting reviews of NHS organizations' arrangements for clinical governance, investigating specific cases of serious service failures and providing advice and guidance on clinical governance.

In 2003, the Healthcare Commission (HCC) was established to replace CHI and incorporates the work of some other commissions. On 1 April 2005, the HCC launched a yearly performance assessment and rating framework for NHS organizations called the 'Annual Health Check'. Through this health check, the HCC measures compliance with the standards of quality set out by the government in the document *Standards for Better Health* (DoH 2004). As a result of this assessment, Trusts are awarded ratings on a four-point scale (excellent, good, fair, or weak) and these are made available publicly. This process of assessment and rating provides an indication to patients and the public of how well NHS organizations are performing.

Clinical audit

Clinical audit is a method for improving health care that involves systematically reviewing clinical practice and recommending changes where necessary. Its aim is to ensure that the best possible care is being delivered to patients and that organizations are actually doing what they think they are doing.

The emergence of clinical audit

The work of Florence Nightingale in the 1850s is generally recognized as one of the earliest examples of clinical audit. By monitoring medical practices during the Crimean War, she was able to identify a link between poor sanitation and high mortality rates. Florence and her team of nurses methodically introduced strict sanitation procedures and were able to report a significant decrease in patient deaths.

Clinical audit (or 'medical audit' as it was known) was not formally introduced as part of professional health care in the NHS until 1989 when the government published its White Paper *Working for Patients* (Department of Health 1989: 3). This paper defines medical audit as 'the systematic critical analysis of the quality of medical care, including the procedures used for diagnosis and treatment, the use of resources, and the resulting outcome and quality of life for the patient'. It also sets out the government's expectation that regular, systematic audit was something in which every doctor would participate. Just a few years later, it became clear that all healthcare professionals, not just hospital doctors, should play an active part in audit and so medical audit evolved into clinical audit. In 1997, the role of clinical audit in the NHS received further significance when the new Labour government introduced clinical governance and identified clinical audit as important to achieving a high-quality NHS (DoH 1997, 1998). The government's commitment to clinical audit was further solidified in 2000 when the *NHS Plan* (Department of Health 2000) established clinical audit as a requirement of all NHS organizations and a mandatory obligation for all doctors employed in, or under contract to the NHS.

The importance of clinical audit in the NHS was highlighted by the public inquiry into children's heart surgery at the Bristol Royal Infirmary (Bristol Royal Infirmary 2001: 455). The inquiry's report recommended that clinical audit 'must be fully supported by Trusts' and 'should be compulsory for all healthcare professionals providing clinical care . . . [The] requirement to participate in it should be included as part of the contract of employment.' Clinical audit is supported by professional bodies as an important part of professional practice. For example, the General Medical Council states that all registered doctors must 'take part in regular and systematic clinical audit' and 'respond constructively to the outcome of audit . . . undertaking further training where necessary' (General Medical Council 2006).

The Health Professions Council's *Standards of Proficiency for Paramedics* (2007) clearly identifies clinical audit as a key obligation and specifies that registrants must 'participate in audit procedures' and 'be able to audit, reflect and review practice'. Therefore, every paramedic has a role to play in clinical audit, whether directly or indirectly.

Link to Chapter 2 to explore the various ethical issues an ambulance clinician may encounter.

What is clinical audit?

Definition of clinical audit

'A quality improvement process that seeks to improve patient care and outcomes through systematic review of care against explicit criteria and the implementation of change' (National Institute for Clinical Excellence 2002: 1).

Clinical audit clearly has an important and prominent role in the NHS, so all healthcare professionals need to have a basic understanding of its principles. To address this requirement for understanding and provide guidance to NHS staff involved in clinical audit, the National Institute for Clinical Excellence (NICE) produced a book called *Principles for Best Practice in Clinical Audit*, where the above definition appeared.

There are many other definitions of clinical audit, but they generally all have the same key elements: the systematic evaluation of practice against criteria and the implementation of change to improve care where indicated. This methodology is widely known as criterion-based clinical audit: criteria are used to assess the quality of care provided by an individual, a team or department, or an entire organization.

The clinical audit process

Clinical audit is a systematic process that consists of an iterative cycle of steps known as the audit cycle (see Figure 4.2). The process involves selecting a topic, setting standards for clinical practice, and then measuring actual practice to determine whether the standards are being met. If practice is shown to deviate from the accepted standard, then causes must be identified and improvements made. After a suitable time interval, clinical practice must be reassessed (reaudited) against the original criteria to confirm an improvement in healthcare delivery. The whole audit process should continue through as many cycles as necessary until there is evidence that improved standards of care are being met and maintained.

Practically any area of clinical care can be selected as a topic for clinical audit, as long at it is measurable. Topic selection will largely be determined at a local level (ideally with input from key stakeholders) and involve a variety of sources including complaints, clinical incident reports and feedback from patient questionnaires or focus groups. The need for a particular clinical audit can also be triggered by the introduction of new drugs or interventions, new guidance or new care pathways. It is also common for topics to be specified at a national level through, for example, National Service Frameworks and NICE guidance. As any audit project will

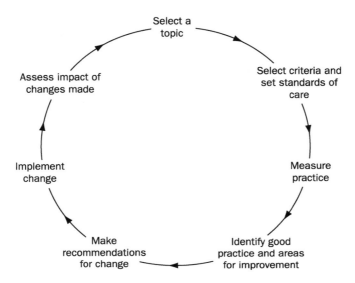

Figure 4.2 The audit cycle

inevitably involve a significant investment of resources, topic selection needs careful consideration and should link in with local and national priorities.

Once a topic has been chosen, the criteria and standards of care must be established. Criteria are essentially explicit statements that describe the aspects of care being measured (for example 'a hospital pre-alert must be placed for patients with cardiac chest pain'). Standards are the expected levels of performance; that is, the amount of times care given should comply with the criteria. Standards are usually expressed as a percentage figure. Criteria and standards of care within UK ambulance services are mainly derived from the Joint Royal Colleges Ambulance Liaison Committee's (JRCALC) *Clinical Practice Guidelines*, although other guidelines are used when relevant.

There are three types of criteria that can be measured:

- Structure – what was needed (e.g. the availability of resources and facilities)?
- Process – what was done/what action was taken (e.g. the treatment given)?
- Outcome – what was the clinical result (e.g. the patient's health status)?

Process criteria are generally considered to be the most sensitive measures of the quality of care, although within the NHS there is growing interest in the use of outcome measures. It is important to use outcome measures with caution as there are often many different factors that contribute to an outcome (such as other treatments and coexisting clinical conditions) and, as such, it is possible that patients who receive a good level of care may experience poor outcomes, and vice versa. Furthermore, some important outcomes occur long after care is provided, so it can be difficult to tease out the direct impact of a particular clinical intervention. This latter limitation is particularly pertinent to ambulance services where patients are frequently handed over to hospitals or other healthcare providers within a relatively short period of time. Outcome measures are also, in practice, very hard to collect (Davies and Crombie 1997). When examining outcomes as part of ambulance service clinical audit, it is often necessary to collect information not only from ambulance service clinical records, but from the records of other organizations that subsequently cared for the patient. With limited resources and authority, ambulance services frequently struggle to obtain data from these different organizations. Nonetheless, despite these limitations, outcome measures can be extremely powerful, particularly when used in conjunction with process measures.

When using outcome criteria, ambulance services may find it less problematic and more useful to select, where practical, outcomes that occur within a short period of time relative to the incident. These would be measured ideally at the point at which the patient is handed over to another healthcare professional and at most within a few days of such handover. In addition to collecting information from the patient care records, outcomes information can be obtained directly from the patient via questionnaires and focus groups. For these techniques to be successful as tools within an audit they must be well structured and the questions must clearly relate to the measures being examined. When using these methods it is essential to consider ethical issues and confidentiality. In some cases approval may be required from a local NHS Research Ethics Committee. When the data has been collected and practice measured, areas of care that do and do not meet the set standards are identified. Where the care given does not meet the set standards, recommendations for improving practice are developed. Once approved by the Trust's relevant executive committees, the recommended changes to practice are implemented in a systematic fashion.

A common criticism of the clinical audit process is that recommended changes are sometimes not fully or effectively implemented. For an audit to succeed in delivering change it is important that there is strong clinical leadership and buy-in at a senior level within the organization. It is also crucial that key stakeholders, including relevant clinicians, patients or service users and staff whose support is necessary to implement changes, are involved from the outset. Key stakeholder involvement ensures that ownership of the project lies with those who are most likely to be affected by its findings. Their involvement also ensures commitment and increases the likelihood that changes to practice, and thus patient care, will be achieved. It is not necessary for all stakeholders to be involved in every stage of the audit, as they can be involved in discrete aspects, such as setting the standards, collecting data or reviewing the results.

Peer review and critical incident analysis

There are a number of common methods of reviewing health care within the NHS, particularly in the hospital setting, that are often mistakenly referred to as clinical audit. Two such examples are peer review and critical incident analysis. Peer review typically involves a group of clinicians randomly selecting a small sample of records for patients who were recently under their care and considering as a group whether the best care was provided. Critical incident analysis usually involves multidisciplinary teams reviewing cases that have caused concern or where there were unexpected, adverse outcomes. These approaches are useful as stand alone methods of assessing performance and highlighting areas of concern. However, when used on their own they do not constitute a clinical audit, as they do not incorporate the full audit cycle. These approaches can form a valuable part of a clinical audit project when incorporated as data collection tools during the measuring practice stage of the audit cycle.

What are the benefits of clinical audit?

Effective clinical audit is vital to the NHS; it brings many benefits to an organization, healthcare professionals, patients and the public. Clinical audit enables organizations and practitioners to demonstrate to themselves and to others the effectiveness and quality of their service. It provides reassurance that patients are receiving the best possible care and can increase confidence in the quality of the service as a whole. Where clinical audit identifies areas for improvement, it can aid practitioners and organizations by pinpointing where further education and training is needed, and so can provide opportunities for learning and development. It can also highlight to organizations areas where new investment and resources are needed to support clinical practices. Most importantly, clinical audit can reduce variability in practice and improve standards of clinical care.

Clinical audit can also provide a valuable contribution to the existing medical evidence base. Using clinical audit findings to add to the evidence base is particularly important in the pre-hospital arena where research evidence for many interventions, although increasing, is currently lacking. Indeed, the findings from ambulance service clinical audits have been used to inform national clinical guidelines. A further, added benefit of clinical audit is that it promotes high standards of clinical record keeping. Clinical audit typically involves extracting information from patient care records and, as such, even when the standard of documentation is not a specific objective of the audit, levels of missing information and other aspects of documentation may be reported and action taken as result to improve levels of documentation.

The role of the ambulance clinician in clinical audit

Every paramedic has a role to play in clinical audit, whether directly or indirectly. Paramedics can undertake their own audit into an area of care that they may consider to be a concern with facilitation and guidance from the trained staff in their Trust's clinical audit department. Alternatively, paramedics can participate in an audit project being run centrally by their clinical audit department. They can contribute in a number of ways, such as assisting with the design of the audit, providing clinical expertise or reviewing selected patient care records. Such direct involvement in clinical audit enables paramedics to actively influence developments in patient care and future clinical practices.

Ambulance clinicians can indirectly contribute to effective clinical audit by ensuring that their patient care records contain a high level of documentation. As in other NHS organizations, ambulance service clinical audit is extremely dependent upon the information documented by the practitioner and the importance of high-quality, complete documentation should not be underestimated. Full and accurate documentation allows those reviewing the records to gain a more comprehensive picture of the care that was delivered, which will in turn lead to accurate decisions about whether or not standards of care were met. Ultimately, without full and accurate documentation, clinical audit cannot accurately assess the real clinical situation and deliver appropriate changes to patient care.

Stop and think – How often are documentation audits carried out in your NHS Trust? Do you understand the importance of your documentation and the link to clinical audit?

Evidence-based practice

Evidence-based practice may be a new term to some paramedics. This is a very brief introduction to the concept of evidence-based practice and further reading will be required in order to fully appreciate and understand the complexities of the process.

Some definitions are included and sources of further reading are clearly identified. Many of the texts are specific to other professions, but the principles of evidence-based practice remain relevant and transferable to paramedic practice.

Definition of quantitative research

Quantitative research produces data that can be expressed statistically (numbers, percentages, tables) and can be subjected to statistical testing. Examples are large-scale social surveys and structured interviews (Marsh and Keating 2006: 735).

Definition of qualitative research

Qualitative research produces data not based on precise statistical measurement, and that is often expressed in words. This style of research encourages understanding and interpretation of experiences. Examples are participant observation and unstructured interviews (Marsh and Keating 2006: 735).

The development of evidence-based practice

The paramedic profession is a relatively new one. If you consider that nursing has a forty-year or so history in terms of research and publication (Craig and Smyth 2007), it is clear that paramedic education is a new concept, so the research of other professions needs to be utilized until paramedic practice has established its own research base. It is not just the quantity but the quality of the research that the paramedic must examine in terms of evidence-based practice. This section of the chapter will provide some key points for the clinician to examine and be aware of when becoming more involved in evidence-based practice.

Evidence-based practice started its journey as 'evidence-based medicine' in the

1980s at a medical school in Canada. It was a term used to describe a 'clinical learning strategy' (Deighan 1996). Sackett *et al.* (2000:1) defined evidence-based medicine as 'the integration of best research evidence with clinical expertise and patient values'. More recent definitions have widened the scope to incorporate other professions and subsequently move away from the term 'medicine' towards 'evidence-based practice'. Muir Gray (1997:18) defined evidence-based practice as 'doing the right things right', where efficiency, quality and 'doing no harm' are central to evidence-based practice. The world of the paramedic is still medically driven in terms of guidelines; the majority of contributors to the JRCALC guidelines are doctors. The challenge to paramedics is to make the patient and patient choice central to their role, incorporating psychology and sociology into the brief, but vital period of time spent caring for the patient.

The use of the term 'caring' has been used specifically, as opposed to 'treating', in order to emphasize the value of your role. After many years' experience in accident and emergency and receiving numerous patients from ambulance crews we have observed that patients who feel 'cared for' are more satisfied with their overall experience. This involves well-developed communication and assessment skills and what you may consider 'small things', like making sure they are comfortable, looking after relatives, explaining what you are doing/what things mean: this is the difference between a caring paramedic and a functional paramedic. Patients recognize the difference.

Steps towards evidence-based practice

Working in a relatively new profession, paramedics may feel that there is not enough research evidence to enable them to know what is 'right' to do in certain circumstances, especially where there are no guidelines/protocols, for instance in the realms of moral and ethical dilemmas. Craig and Smyth (2007: 7) advocate that 'the ethos of evidence-based practice should stop us in our tracks to reflect on the impact of what we are doing'. Craig and Smyth (2007) believe reflective practice is a key component of evidence-based health care.

Link to Chapter 5 to establish further links between reflection and evidence-based practice.

Boxes 4.1 and 4.2 provide a very brief overview of the 'things to consider' when developing evidence-based practice.

Box 4.1 highlights the key skills regarded as fundamental to begin to develop the skills of working in a more evidence-based manner; these are expanded upon in the following paragraphs. The process of evidence-based practice stems from the question asked. Asking questions is a skill; questions need to be phrased in order to obtain a meaningful answer. This applies to asking questions of research, as well as asking

---

Box 4.1 Skills required and steps to be taken by the practitioner in order to embrace evidence-based practice

- How to ask the right question:

    - clarify what information is required
    - take time to develop questions in order to get the information you need.

- Searching the literature

    - developing more advanced searching techniques will enhance your search and results
    - systematic review can take many formats, depending on the audience they are written for. For example, chapters in textbooks, reports to expert committees and reviews for clinical journals.

- Critical appraisal of quantitative studies:

    - is the quality of the study good enough for you to use the findings?
    - can the evidence be applied in your clinical setting?

- Qualitative research

    - develop your skills of critical appraisal.

- Integrating research evidence into clinical decisions. Consider:

    - clinical expertise
    - patient preferences, values and beliefs
    - limited resources for health care.

(Craig and Smyth 2007)

---

questions directly to people (Craig 2007). Ambulance clinicians ask questions in the course of their working lives. The following case study may help explain the value of asking the right question.

Case study

A clinician attends a patient who has tripped and fallen onto an open fire. The patient has sustained a laceration to his forearm from the fireplace and also has a burn to his hand and wrist. The clinician would ask herself, 'What dressing should I apply to this wound/injury?'

Whilst the clinician might have a preferred clinical approach to this situation, there should be evidence available in order to answer this question. This evidence will not necessarily be available 'on the road' but further investigation at some point will benefit future interactions with patients suffering similar injuries.

An ambulance clinician working in an evidence-based practice manner will then evaluate the evidence for its validity and usefulness. These findings are then used in clinical situations, taking into consideration patient needs and available resources, to achieve a course of action and decision making. Ambulance clinicians should always evaluate their performance and the outcome of the decision they have taken (Craig 2007). In order to evaluate any evidence, the clinician must first develop literature-searching skills.

Ambulance clinicians' skill at literature searching will depend on their exposure to education and level of educational achievement. Before anyone can develop advanced searching techniques, as recommended in Box 4.1, they may require help to achieve basic searching principles. Higher education libraries will have literature, leaflets or classes to help students develop these fundamental skills. These skills are also essential for sourcing articles for academic coursework, so are worthwhile and lifelong skills to take time to develop and understand.

Definition of critical appraisal

Critical appraisal is defined by O'Rourke (2005) as 'a discipline for increasing the effectiveness of your reading, by encouraging systematic assessment of reports of research evidence to see which ones can best answer clinical problems and inform *best practice*'.

In order to appraise quantitative and qualitative studies critically, the above definition must be understood. Gibson and Glenny (2007) suggest that the process of critical appraisal can be extrapolated into three parts, as represented in Figure 4.3.

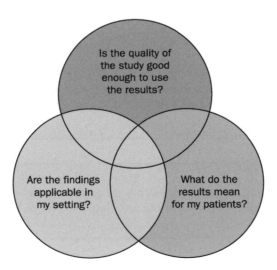

Figure 4.3 The three aspects of critical appraisal for evidence-based practice (Gibson and Glenny 2007)

How can you decide if the quality of the study is good enough? Both researchers and clinicians have worked hard to develop toolkits or checklists to help the novice researcher or clinician ascertain the quality of studies. Once these toolkits or checklists are accessed and the necessary skills acquired, the clinician must consider if they have clinical expertise. Miles *et al.* (2000) describe some of the main characteristics of competent clinical practice; see the definition below.

Definition of competent practice

Miles *et al.* (2000) believe that competent practice relies not only on the findings derived from scientific research, such as large population studies or qualitative research, but also on the practitioner's intuition, common sense and a clear understanding and knowledge of the meaning that the situation has for the patient and their family.

Competent practice and clinical expertise are different. The work of Benner (1984) is seminal when discussing the development of the practitioner from novice to expert. Benner (1984) describes several stages:

Novice → Advanced → Competent → Proficient → Expert
            beginner   practitioner   practitioner

These stages are inextricably linked to the belief that clinical expertise has a direct relation to the length of exposure to practice. This obviously relies on clinicians recalling and reflecting upon their experiences in practice. Benner's (1984) definition of expertise clearly refers to this process.

Definition of expertise

Benner (1984: 294) believes expertise develops through '. . . a process of comparing whole similar and dissimilar clinical situations with one another, so the expert has deep background understanding of the clinical situations based upon many past paradigm cases . . .'

Link to Chapter 5 for more details on how to make patient encounters more meaningful and good learning experiences. Link to Chapter 14 for theories on how decisions are made.

It must be remembered that, as with any human, even experts may not always make the correct clinical decision. There are other issues to be considered; the importance of taking into account the patient's values and wishes must not be negated. With more and more people living with chronic illnesses in the UK, the clinician can also learn from patients and their families. Patients with experience of living with a condition are often called 'expert patients'. These patients know what works for them and their condition. They live with the condition; many of them contribute to the Department of Health's National Service Frameworks for their specific condition and the sensible clinician will be open to learning from such patients. The amalgamation of both the clinician's knowledge and the patient's expertise, in terms of his life and condition, should make for a comprehensive, holistic and highly satisfactory healthcare encounter for both parties.

In addition to the skills described on the previous few pages, there are a number of ways in which evidence presents itself to the practitioner (Craig and Smyth 2007). In order to use available evidence, the paramedic should be aware of the variety of evidence bases (Craig and Smyth 2007): see Table 4.1.

Range of evidence bases

Table 4.1 Range of evidence bases relevant to paramedic practice

Type of evidence base	Example
Public health intervention	Legislation concerning the compulsory wearing of seat belts
Health-related behaviours	Anti-smoking campaign – realizing that alternatives need to be in place (nicotine patches, support groups), rather than just presenting evidence that smoking is detrimental to health. Considering 'patient perspectives' is the key to evidence-based practice (Sackett *et al.* 2000).
Paramedic interventions	Drawing upon sources of evidence to make decisions about interventions, such as giving medication and what observations to undertake.
Communication	Quality ambulance clinician care is often determined by effective communication, not just treating and transferring the patient safely. Again the consideration of patient perspectives is very important.
Management evidence	The paramedic will find herself in the position of managing a team, albeit a small team. The proposals of the consultation document *Direction of Travel for Urgent Care* (DoH 2006), due as a White Paper in Spring 2007, may signal the way forward for more teams of multi-professionals to work in the community (as already occurs in some areas). The paramedic may be in a position to manage these teams. In these circumstances, it is vital that the paramedic utilizes the wide evidence base within management sciences in order to be more effective in managerial roles.

Stop and think – Consider the range of evidence bases in Box 4.1 and think about which ones are used more frequently in the course of your daily activities.

Developing an evidence-based culture

Once the paramedic has identified the range of evidence bases, and identified and refined the skills to move towards evidence-based practice, the process of implementation has to be carefully considered, planned and evaluated. The realities of practice may mean that practitioners encounter resistance to change; a change in culture within the organization maybe required. It is important for paramedics to explore how they can contribute to an organizational change and a shift in culture towards evidence-based practice.

Link to the clinical audit section of this chapter (pages 43–8) to establish how evidence-based practice and clinical audit are inextricably linked.

Link to Chapter 3 to explore the value of effective communication to evidence-based practice.

Link to Chapter 15 to read about strategies that may be useful when attempting to change practice.

Box 4.2 How can an evidence-based culture be developed?

1 Diagnosing challenges to changing practice – understanding the complexity of organizations at all levels, national (Department of Health) and local (local NHS Trust).

2 How can evidence-based innovation and culture be encouraged?

Need to take into account the:
   i)   innovation
   ii) individuals and groups involved
   iii) system in which the innovator must operate.

3 How can change happen?
   i)   developing evidence-based literature
   ii) identifying what works and what does not
   iii) understanding and utilizing change models.

(Craig and Smyth 2007)

> **Stop and think** – How can you become involved in supporting the development of evidence-based practice in your NHS Trust? Are there any working groups, committees or research projects you might be interested in joining?

Evidence-based practice may not be as simple as it sounds (Craig and Smyth 2007). Paramedics are in a prime position to research numerous areas of their own practice and contribute to a research base on which the future development of the profession will build. It is, therefore, exceptionally important that paramedics take time to explore the key aspects of evidence-based practice and to build solid foundations that will stand the test of time. Until paramedics are conversant with the research attributes required to ensure their work is truly evidence-based it maybe desirable to work with research and academic colleagues as part of their own continuing professional development.

Conclusion

This chapter has highlighted some important areas of practice that have their roots in providing a quality service. It is hoped that the various sections have improved your knowledge and understanding of the purposes of each aspect and that you will wish to investigate further. Quality of care given to patients is paramount and should be the aim of all clinicians.

Chapter key points

- The issues discussed within this chapter affect ambulance clinicians practice, either explicitly or implicitly. They are all closely related.
- Clinical audit is undertaken across all healthcare environments and the outcome often influences practice at a later date.
- All patients deserve a practitioner who is aware of anti-discriminatory practice and practices within these guidelines at all times. The practitioner's behaviour and attitudes can influence a patient's future decision on whether or not to access health care.
- All practice is influenced and guided by evidence-based practice; it is important for the ambulance clinician to understand the theory and development behind such practice.

References, suggested reading and useful websites

Benner, P. (1984) *From Novice to Expert: Excellence and Power in Clinical Nursing Practice.* Menro Park CA: Addison-Wesley.

Bristol Royal Infirmary Inquiry (2001) *Learning from Bristol: The Report of the Public Inquiry into Children's Heart Surgery at the Bristol Royal Infirmary 1984–1995.* London: The Stationery Office. www.bristol-inquiry.org.uk/final_report/the_report.pdf. (Accessed 23 January 2007.)

Craig, J.V. (2007) How to ask the right question, in J.V. Craig and R.L. Smyth (2007) *The Evidence-based Practice Manual for Nurses*. Section 2. London: Churchill Livingstone/ Elsevier.

Craig, J.V. and Smyth, R.L. (2007) *The Evidence-based Practice Manual for Nurses*. London: Churchill Livingstone/Elsevier.

Davies, H.T.O. and Crombie, I.K. (1997) Interpreting health outcomes, *Journal of Evaluation Clinical Practice*, 3(3):187–200.

Deighan, M. (1996) Defining evidence-based health care: a health-care learning strategy?, *NT Research*, 1(5): 332–9.

DoH (Department of Health) (1989) *Working for Patients*, Cm 555. London: HMSO.

DoH (1997) *The New NHS: Modern, Dependable*, Cm 3807. London: HMSO.

DoH (1998) *A First Class Service: Quality in the NHS*. www.dh.gov.uk/PublicationsAnd Statistics/Publications/PublicationsPolicyAndGuidance/ PublicationsPolicyAndGuidanceArticle/fs/en?CONTENT_ID=4006902&chk=j2Tt7C. (Accessed 23 January 2007.)

DoH (1999a) *Clinical Governance: Quality in the New NHS*, Health Service Circular, 1999/065. www.dh.gov.uk/assetRoot/04/01/20/43/04012043.pdf. (Accessed 29 January 2007.)

DoH (1999b) *Health Act*. London: HMSO.

DoH (2000) *The NHS Plan: A Plan For Investment, A Plan For Reform*, Cm 4818-I. London: HMSO.

DoH (2004) *Standards for Better Health*. www.dh.gov.uk/assetRoot/04/08/66/66/04086666.pdf. (Accessed 23 January 2007.)

DoH (2006) *Direction of Travel for Urgent Care: A Discussion Document*. London: The Stationery Office.

Donaldson, L.J. (2000) Clinical governance: a mission to improve, *British Journal of Clinical Governance*, 5(1): 6–8.

Donaldson, L.J. and Gray, J.A.M. (1998) Clinical governance: a quality duty for health organisations, *Quality in Health Care*, 7(Suppl.): S37–S44.

General Medical Council (2006) http://www.gmc-uk.org/guidance/good_medical_practice/ maintaining_good_medical_practice/performance.asp. (Accessed 23 January 2007.)

Gibson, F. and Glenny, A.M. (2007) Critical appraisal of quantitative studies 1: Is the quality of the study good enough for you to use the findings?, in J.V. Craig and R.L. Smyth (2007) *The Evidence-based Practice Manual for Nurses*. London: Churchill Livingstone/ Elsevier.

Health Professions Council (2007) *Standards of Proficiency for Paramedics*. www.hpc-uk.org/ publications/standards/index.asp?id=48. (Accessed 23 January 2007.)

Marsh, I. and Keating, M. (2006) *Sociology. Making Sense of Society*, 3rd edn. Pearson Education Limited. London: Prentice-Hall.

Miles, A., Charlton, B., Bentley, P., Polychronis, A., and Grey, J. (2000) New perspectives in the evidence-based healthcare debate, *Journal of Evaluation in Clinical Practice*, 6: 77–84.

Muir Gray, J.A. (1997) *Evidence-based Health Care. How to Make Health Policy and Management Decisions*. London: Churchill Livingstone.

National Audit Office (2003) *Achieving Improvements through Clinical Governance. A Progress Report on Implementation by NHS Trusts*. London: The Stationery Office.

National Institute for Clinical Excellence (2002) *Principles for Best Practice in Clinical Audit*. London: Radcliffe Medical Press Ltd.

Oliver, M. (1996) *Understanding Disability: From Theory to Practice*. London: Macmillan.

O'Rourke, A. (2005) Critical appraisal, in A. Bowling and S. Ebrahim (eds) *Handbook of Health Research Methods: Investigation, Measurement and Analysis*. Buckingham: Open University Press.

Oxford University Press (2006) *Concise Oxford English Dictionary*. Oxford: Oxford University Press.

Oyebode, F., Brown, N. and Parry, L. (1999a) Clinical governance in practice, *Advances in Psychiatric Treatment*, 5: 399–404.

Oyebode, F., Brown, N. and Parry, E. (1999b) Clinical governance: application to psychiatry, *Psychiatric Bulletin*, 23: 7–10.

Sackett, D.L., Strauss, S.E., Richardson, W.S., Rosenberg, W. and Haynes, R.B. (2000) *Evidence-based Medicine: How to Practise and Teach EBM*. London: Churchill Livingstone.

Thompson, N. (2002) *People Skills*, 2nd edn. Basingstoke: Palgrave Macmillan.

Thompson, N. (2003) *Promoting Equality. Challenging Discrimination and Oppression*, 2nd edn. Basingstoke: Palgrave Macmillan.

Thompson, N. (2006) *Anti-discriminatory Practice*, 4th edn. Basingstoke: Palgrave Macmillan publishing in conjunction with the British Association of Social Workers.

5

Reflective practice in relation to pre-hospital care
Amanda Blaber

Topics covered:

- Introduction
- Why is this relevant?
- How do I decide what to write about?
- Making reflection more structured
- Uses of reflection
- Explanation of Gibbs's model of reflection
- The value of reflective writing within portfolio/profile development
- Conclusion
- Chapter key points
- References and suggested reading

Introduction

Every day most people sit and think about what has happened to them during the day. This can take several forms: personal thought with no verbal communication, talking over your day, discussing things with loved ones and/or friends, talking on the telephone and talking to anyone who will listen – pets are useful here! Discussion may also occur with colleagues about specific incidents/occurrences during the shift/day.

Definition of reflective practice

Bolton (2001: 4) defines the term reflective practice as 'a process of learning and developing through examining our own practice, opening our practice to scrutiny by others, and studying texts from the wider sphere. It is a focusing closer and closer.'

Why is this relevant?

Ambulance clinicians encounter many incidents and have many experiences during episodes of care with patients and colleagues. At the time it may not be appropriate to review the call or to reflect on the experience. This chapter includes some useful models and strategies to assist the clinician to make sense of and learn from the experience. This can only benefit clinicians' professional development and future patient care.

How do I decide what to write about?

We may sit and think about our day, but when we are asked to think of 'something' to reflect upon we often struggle. Rolfe *et al.* (2001) describe the term critical incident as being the 'something' we are looking for. The development of the term critical incident originates from John Flanagan, a psychologist working within the American Air Force in the 1950s. It is a popular misconception by health professionals that the term critical incident relates specifically to large and highly dramatic incidents; this could not be further from Flanagan's definition:

> By an incident is meant any observable human activity that is sufficiently complete in itself to permit inferences and predictions to be made about the person performing the act. To be critical, an incident must occur in a situation where the purpose or intent of the act seems fairly clear to the observer and where its consequences are sufficiently definite to leave little doubt concerning its effects.
>
> (Flanagan 1954: 327)

It is clear from Flanagan's (1954) definition that he intended the term 'critical incident' to refer to small occurrences, as well as large events. In terms of health care, sometimes we do not see the consequences of our actions or non-actions, as Flanagan (1954) suggests. If we are taking Flanagan's definition literally, when choosing an incident to reflect upon, we often cannot satisfy the second part of the definition ('where its consequences are sufficiently definite to leave little doubt concerning its effects'), so we may require another guide to help us make appropriate choices for reflection.

The work of Atkins and Murphy (1993) identifies stages of the reflective process, as seen in Box 5.1. The definition explaining how an individual chooses to reflect on

Box 5.1 Stages of the reflective process	
Stage 1	An awareness of uncomfortable feelings and thoughts
Stage 2	A critical analysis of the situation, which is constructive and involves an examination of feelings and knowledge
Stage 3	Development of a new perspective on the situation
	(Atkins and Murphy 1993)

an incident is provided by Atkins and Murphy (1993) and is very different to that of Flanagan (1954): 'An awareness of uncomfortable feelings or thoughts. This arises from a realization that, in a situation, the knowledge one was applying was not sufficient in itself to explain what was happening in that unique situation' (Atkins and Murphy 1993: 50). This definition clearly refers to negative feelings as the stimulus for choice of reflective writing. This is not always the case, but may be useful for the student who is trying to choose subjects for reflective writing for the first time. It is also vital to reflect on our positive experiences in practice and reflect on what made the experience/situation so good, in order that we can repeat it on a consistent basis. As Rolfe *et al.* (2001: 58, added emphasis) assert, reflection can be about 'anything that happens to us that *we want to write about for some reason*'.

Once you have the experience that you wish to write about, you need to think about how to structure your thoughts, in order to learn.

Making reflection more structured

Reflection is, therefore, nothing to be scared of – we all 'do it' every day in one form or another. In order for any experience to be used as a learning tool, reflection requires structure. Otherwise your thoughts and discussions may not reach a conclusion or be evaluated and may be left as a *moan* (if the experience was not a good one) or as a *celebration* of your success (if the experience was good). Indeed, reflective writing can be about anything at all (Rolfe *et al.* 2001). Schön (1983) differentiates between reflection that happens as you are practising, defining this as reflection *in action*, and reflection *upon action*, which is the consideration of events after their occurrence, so that practice can be enhanced effectively in the future. This chapter is concerned with reflecting on events after they have occurred, so the focus is on reflection upon action. Once the experience/event has occurred what can you *do* with it?

Uses of reflection

A model of reflection provides a structure for you to follow, in order that you can make some sense of what happened. It also enables you to highlight what you might need to learn or practise, if the experience involved the practice of a skill or communication with a patient/relative, for instance. On a more positive note, reflection also facilitates examination of an experience where everything went very well, for example the patient received a high standard of care in a timely manner by a cohesive team. In circumstances like these it is also valuable to reflect on what *fell into place* to make the experience go so well, by exploring all aspects of the experience, such as

- the circumstances of the call;
- characteristics and behaviour of the patient and family;
- communications: what was said, how it was said;
- what was done for the patient and how it was done;
- who were the people involved;

- how they got on together;
- what were their characteristics, and so on.

Some of these points, if reflected upon, may give you a gold standard that you wish to aspire to in future calls of the same nature. There may be certain aspects that you can replicate on future calls, for example your communication strategies, and involvement of family members. By reflecting on situations that have gone well and not so well, you are continually exploring your own practice and learning from patients, families, colleagues and peers. This can only be good for your continuing professional development. So reflection should never cease. It also has a role to play in maintaining our own mental well-being as healthcare professionals.

> Link to Chapter 16 to read about the importance of reviewing practice issues.

 Stop and think – How many times have you woken in the middle of the night *going over* something that has happened at work?

Very often a situation that is not reflected upon will 'creep up on you' and 'play on your mind'. For most situations in the realms of our normal daily workload, reflection may prevent many a sleepless night. Depending on the nature of the situation/experience, reflection will not be sufficient and other strategies, such as counselling, may be more appropriate. Try it.

> Link to Chapter 8, pages 115–16, in order to recognize signs and symptoms of post-traumatic stress disorder.

Explanation of Gibbs's model of reflection

Figure 5.1 provides a description of one of the many models of reflection. Gibbs (1988) may be described as simplistic and that is exactly why it is a good model to start with. Once you are 'grabbed' by the reflective 'bug' you may find other models that you prefer or that are more useful in certain circumstances. Reflection is very often a personal experience, so not all of us will like using the same model. Each section of Figure 5.1 has some questions that you may find useful to explain how you may want to structure your thinking, in order to get the most from the reflective experience. You may wish to mentally work through your experience, or at other times you may be required to write a reflective account for your academic studies. Rowland (1993) values writing as a way of sharing, expressing, assessing and developing professional practice. Writing about your experiences is different from talking about an experience. Bolton (2001) believes that writing enables contact with thoughts and ideas that the writer did not know she had. It also facilitates understanding between theory and practice and enables the writer to make connections that would otherwise not have been made (Rolfe *et al.* 2001).

Figure 5.1 represents a modified Gibbs (1988) cycle and draws upon the work of other reflective writers to provide some questions that should assist you in the reflective process (Gibbs 1988; Jasper 2003; Palmer *et al.* 2004). Sometimes the hardest part of the process is finding something you want to reflect upon and then getting started. This structure should help you.

The value of reflective writing within portfolio/profile development

Both the Health Professions Council (2007) and British Paramedic Association (2006) suggest that all registered paramedics commence and maintain a personal portfolio or profile whilst registered. This is also the practice for other healthcare professions and recommendations from registrant bodies. Writing for your portfolio/ profile has different connotations to writing for an assessment. Jasper (1999) has developed a model to show the ways in which reflective writing can enhance your professional practice. It has equal resonance for any healthcare professional involved in patient care (see Figure 5.2).

The model, Figure 5.2, examines professional practice in terms of four categories and lists the learning activities/requirements in order to develop professional practice. These four categories have also been useful for healthcare professionals engaged in clinical supervision and provide a clear structure when considering or discussing an experience or client case study. On an individual level, Rolfe *et al.* (2001) suggest that this model is useful for focusing reflective writing within portfolios.

Link to the critical thinking skills section, Chapter 14, to consider critical thinking and the characteristics of a critical thinker, in terms of reflecting upon an incident or experience.

Describe the situation
What happened?
Who was involved? Where were you?
What were you doing?
What was your part in the situation?
What were other people doing?
What was the result of the situation?

Action plan for the future
How might you be able to use this
   learning in the future in the same
   or similar situations?
How will you act differently if the
   same or similar situation arose again?
From what you have learnt, what can
   you apply to other situations?

**Discuss your feelings about the
   situation**
How were you feeling when the
   event started?
What were you thinking at the time?
How did the situation make you feel?
What did other people's words
   make you think?
How did this make you feel?
How did you feel about the outcome
   of the situation?
What emotions did you go through
   during the situation?
Which is the most important or
   significant feeling/emotion for you
   and why?

**Draw some conclusions about the
   situation and what you have learnt from it**
How could you have improved the situation
   for yourself, the patient or others involved?
What could you have done differently?
What have you learnt from this situation?

Evaluate and analyse the situation
What was good about the situation?
What was bad, difficult, problematic about the situation?
What went well?
What did you do well?
What did others do well?
Did you expect anything different to happen, if so what and why?
What went wrong, or did not turn out the way you expected?
In what way did you contribute to the situation, either positively
   or negatively?
What knowledge from theory and research can you apply to
   the situation?
Find it, use it and reference it within this section to either dispute
   what happened or substantiate your view/actions.
What broader issues e.g. ethical, political, legal or social arise
   from this situation?
Has this situation changed the way you think you will act in similar
   situations in the future?

Figure 5.1 Reflective practice diagram
Source: Adapted from: Gibbs (1988); Jasper (2003); Palmer *et al.* (2004)

Professional development
Developing a knowledge base
Evidence of professional practice
Evidence-based practice

Critical thinking
Making connections
Organizing thoughts/structure
Taking a new perspective on issues
Exploring issues

**DEVELOPING EVIDENCE OF
ACCOUNTABLE PROFESSIONAL
PRACTICE**

Personal development
Development tool
Learning from experience
Cognitive, deliberative process
Developing analytical skills

Outcomes for clinical practice
Moving care forward
Delivering the best patient care

Figure 5.2 A model of the way that experienced nurses use reflective writing in their professional practice
Source: Jasper (1999)

Conclusion

By answering, or at least considering all or most of the questions in Figure 5.1, you will be reflecting in a meaningful manner. You may discover aspects of your *self* during the process which may surprise, concern or please you. True reflection is an honest process; you should try to be open to these possibilities. Learning about us, examining the actions of ourselves and others is all part of the process and at times maybe uncomfortable. Persevere and if you improve the care or the way one person is cared for in the pre-hospital environment then the process of reflection has been worthwhile and you have learnt from your experiences.

Chapter key points

- Reflective practice has many purposes, ranging through personal self-awareness, professional development, reviewing practice issues and improvement of patient care.
- There are a wide variety of strategies and models that a clinician may find useful when embracing reflective practice.
- Reflective practice also plays an important role in helping ambulance clinicians to maintain their own positive mental health by encouraging thought and analysis when considering more emotional and difficult calls/jobs.

References and suggested reading

Atkins, S. and Murphy, K. (1993) Reflective practice, *Nursing Standard*, 8 (39): 49–54.
Bolton, G. (2001) *Reflective Practice: Writing and Professional Development*. London: Paul Chapman Publishing.
British Paramedic Association (2006) *Curriculum Framework for Ambulance Education*. London: BPA.

Flanagan, J. (1954) The critical incident technique, *Psychological Bulletin*, 51 (4): 327–58.

Gibbs, G. (1988) *Learning by Doing: A Guide to Teaching and Learning Methods*. Oxford: Further Education Unit, Oxford Polytechnic.

Health Professions Council (2007) *Standards of Proficiency for Paramedics*. www.hpc-uk.org/ publications/standards/index.asp?id=48. (Accessed 23 January 2007.)

Jasper, M.A. (1999) Assessing and improving student outcomes through reflective writing, in C. Rust (ed.) *Improving Student Learning – Improving Student Learning Outcomes*. Oxford: Oxford Centre for Staff Development.

Jasper, M. (2003) *Beginning Reflective Practice*. Cheltenham: Nelson Thornes.

Palmer, P., Burns, S. and Bulman, C. (2004) *Reflective Practice in Nursing: The Growth of the Professional Practitioner*. Oxford: Blackwell Scientific.

Rolfe, G., Freshwater, D. and Jasper, M. (2001) *Critical Reflection for Nursing and the Helping Professions*. Basingstoke: Palgrave Macmillan.

Rowland, S. (1993) *The Enquiring Tutor*. Lewes: Falmer.

Schön, D.A. (1983) *The Reflective Practitioner: How Professionals Think in Action*. New York: Basic Books.

6

Psychology: an introduction
Jackie Whitnell

Topics covered:

- Introduction
- Why is this topic relevant?
- Psychology – what is it?
- Different approaches to psychology
- Conclusion
- Chapter key points
- References, suggested reading and useful website

Introduction

Have you ever considered someone's actions and thought to yourself

- Why did they do that?
- How does that make me feel about their action?
- What were they thinking of?
- I knew they were going to do/say that?

That's psychology – the study of behaviour and mental processes. As you read more about psychology you will be amazed at the number of different approaches that psychologists adopt in their attempt to gain a greater understanding of human behaviour. Some approaches appear similar, such as cognitivism and learning theory (otherwise know as behaviourism – indeed, cognitivism found its origins in

---

ψ (This symbol is the Greek letter 'psi', often used as an abbreviation for the word 'Psychology'.)
It is the 23rd letter of the Greek alphabet. Pronounced as si (sigh).

behaviourism); however, some approaches are very different. This chapter will endeavour to provide the reader with an introduction to psychology.

Why is this topic relevant?

Psychology, the understanding of behaviour and mental processes of the human being, is a core subject for the ambulance clinician and healthcare professionals as it serves to underpin their understanding of health and health behaviours.

In order that ambulance clinicians and healthcare professionals can help patients/clients who are ill or disabled it is important that they understand how humans function when they are healthy. To work successfully in the healthcare profession you will need an understanding of not only how people function but also how they interact with each other. There are many reasons why psychology is relevant to health care; it is useful to help understand the needs of not only the individual, but also groups of people. It is especially useful to understand those that are potentially vulnerable including babies, children, the mentally ill and elderly plus those that have a disability or learning needs, amongst many others. As a healthcare professional you will spend many working days caring for those who experience social/economic disadvantage and those who cannot cope with life. You will be aware that in today's society people are living longer and with chronic illness and life-limiting conditions, so an understanding of behaviour and mental processes can help in the care of such people. Psychology also informs us of individual patterns of behaviour and aids our understanding of the difficulties with behaviour change (Hewstone *et al.* 2006).

Psychology – what is it?

There are many factors that determine our behaviour, for example:

- the genes we are born with;
- our physiological system (brain, nervous system, endocrine system);
- our cognitive system (thoughts, perception, memory);
- the social and cultural environments in which we develop over time;
- our life experiences including those from childhood;
- our personal and individual differences including our IQ, personality and mental health.

Stop and think – A man punches another man outside a public house in an attack of aggressive behaviour. How do we understand that behaviour? Could it be that:

- the attacker has inherited his genes from his parents and his father is known for his short temper (genetics and physiology);
- the attacker experienced violence in his childhood in his family home (learned behaviour);

- he has a history of personality disorder and is experiencing mental health problems (social/cultural experiences);
- the attacker was frustrated with the other person and this gave him thoughts of anger and aggression (cognitivism);
- in a social situation the attacker thought the other person was insulting his family and in his culture it is acceptable to defend his family in that way (social/cultural)?

Psychology is not simply common sense! It is an enormous subject and the knowledge of psychology can be usefully applied in many different professions and walks of life. For the purpose of this chapter, psychology will be considered in brief to provide the reader with a thirst for further exploration of knowledge. As previously stated, psychology is the study of behaviour and mental processes and different schools of thought within psychology place differing degrees of emphasis on understanding these different approaches. Psychology is not a single subject; rather it is a coalition of different specialisms (Berryman *et al.* 2006).

The different schools of thought are many and include: developmental, cognitive, biological, social, health, occupational and clinical psychology, to name but a few. This introductory textbook will include a sequence of three chapters on psychology: an overview of psychology (this chapter), Developmental Psychology, which will consider the theoretical perspectives of child development (Chapter 7) and Abnormal Psychology, a discussion on mental health issues (Chapter 8). This text will also include discussion of atypical development in children (included in Chapter 7) and the important aspect of 'safeguarding children' (Chapter 9). These areas have been chosen not because they are essentially more important than others but because ambulance clinicians and allied health professionals in their day-to-day working life will benefit from an understanding of the theoretical underpinning around these topics, thus linking theory to practice.

Psychology is an academic discipline, one which emerged as a distinct discipline approximately 150 years ago. It has its roots in physiology, physics and philosophy and is a discipline which relies on theories to understand how people behave and think and attempts to make predictions about how processes, such as memory, will occur. In order to do this, psychologists design and undertake carefully planned experiments and observations and use specific scientific methods to collect data, which after careful analysis enables them to make such predictions. However, theories are ever evolving and psychologists may modify them over time when they continue to research their chosen approach/es further (Hewstone *et al.* 2006).

Psychology is characterized by a number of different theoretical approaches to the behaviour and mental functioning of individuals. A theory is based on a set of facts, principles and generalizations that explains development, generates hypotheses and provides a coherent framework for future research. It connects facts and observation, putting the details of life into a meaningful whole. Psychologists are extraordinary intellectual leaders/researchers who have fashioned the framework over time and as a result have developed theories on the topic of psychology. Theorists have many different viewpoints. Some approaches that are conspicuous in current psychology are psychodynamic, learning theory, cognitivism and humanism. Within this chapter we will consider these in the broad sense and then further on in Chapter 7, in relation to developmental psychology. Chapter 6 will also consider, albeit briefly, alternative perspectives on psychology to that of the mainstream: psychobiological, social cultural and social constructivism. For further reading on these approaches the reader would be advised to refer to general psychology texts, such as Zimbardo *et al.* (1995); Eysenck (2000); Gross (2001); Atkinson *et al.* (2003); and Hewstone *et al.* (2006).

Psychology is concerned with human beings, but what makes a human a person is subject to much debate. Questions have been asked as to whether a person is a product of pre-wiring (according to laws of nature) or develops from a person's nurturing environment (laws of behaviour) in that they are a product of creativity, free willed and responsible for their own actions. This question has, over decades, been transposed into what is commonly called the 'nature/nurture' debate. This is the long-standing debate among philosophers, psychologists and educators concerning the importance of heredity and learning. On the one hand, historically, philosophers believed the human infant is born without knowledge and skills (a blank slate or 'tabula rasa') – this is an empiricist viewpoint. This perspective argues that human development occurs as the person is nurtured through observation and experiences (Greek 'empeiria' literally means 'experience'). This viewpoint argues that all hypotheses about human functioning should have an observable consequence, which can be confirmed or refuted by data collection and statistical testing. An opposing view from a nativist's perspective argues that nature, heredity and genes pre-wire us and this subsequently shapes our development. Based on the work of many, current thinking holds with the view that the thoughts of empiricists and nativists do injustice to the richness of human functioning. Moreover, today investigators are more interested in how nature and nurture interact and the importance of both for development (Berryman *et al.* 2006; Hewstone *et al.* 2006).

Theoretical perspectives also vary in terms of the time span that psychologists consider, for example psychologists including Freud consider past experiences to explain present behaviour, including experiences in childhood, abuse and family break-up (Freud). Or the focus could be on the present, observing behaviour here and now (Skinner) and how the behaviour is shaped by reward and reinforcement (operant conditioning). This chapter continues with a brief introduction to four main approaches in psychology. These approaches will be considered further in relation to developmental psychology in the following chapter.

Different approaches to psychology

Psychodynamic approach

Sigmund Freud (1856–1939) is a name that often springs to mind when people think of psychology. Freud studied how unconscious inner forces (id, ego and super ego) purportedly produce urges and wishes that drive our behaviour. Freud was credited for making the unconscious worthy of serious inquiry. His techniques (used on people who had mental health problems), termed psychoanalysis, were that of free association and dream analysis. He believed that these techniques led him to an understanding of the patient's problems and by bringing that source out in the open, into conscious awareness, the emotional release (or catharsis) would assist in helping the patient towards a solution to the problem. However, he has been criticized for his theory being that of mythology, drama and legend as opposed to sound empirical theory. Freud's ideas and evidence are open to many differing interpretations and cannot be tested or verified in the way that modern psychology believes to be essential (Atkinson *et al.* 2003). However, Freud's views of the human mind and behaviour have influenced psychological thinking over time, although they are not central to it.

Definitions of psychoanalytical terms

Psychoanalysis: Freud's theory of human behaviour and the treatment he devised for mental disorders.

Id: The id works in accord with the pleasure principle. The id is the part of the unconscious mind containing the sexual instinct (libido). Emphasis is on immediate satisfaction.

Ego: The ego is the conscious, rational mind; this develops in the first two years of life. It works with what is happening in the real world.

Superego: This develops around 5 years of age and is concerned with moral issues. The child adopts many of the same-sexed parent's values.

Defence mechanisms: These are strategies used by the ego to defend itself against anxiety.

Learning theory (Behaviourism)

First developed in the United States in 1912, its origins lie in animal research which was mainly concerned with understanding the processes of learning under highly controlled conditions. Learning theory argues that the process of learning can be defined as that which has occurred when a relatively permanent change in behaviour or behaviour potential has been produced by experience. Watson, Pavlov and Skinner from 1912 onwards were influential theorists who dedicated their studies to observable behaviour. They argued that our capacity for learning depends on both genetic heritage and the nature of our environment. The study of learning has been dominated by the behaviourist approach, as represented in their work. Two main areas of study are that of classical conditioning and operant conditioning.

Link to Chapter 7 for further discussion on conditioning.

Cognitivism

Cognitivism found its origins in learning theory with emphasis on controlled observation of behaviour but with different considerations, such as how people think, make decisions and so on.

Since the inception of computers, researchers such as Broadbent (1958) examined the ways in which people mentally process information. The term cognitivism usually refers to mental representation of events, to the process of interpretation, prediction and evaluation of the environment, as well as to beliefs, thoughts and expectations (Hewstone *et al.* 2006). The so-called 'cognitive revolution' has emerged over the past few decades as a direct challenge to learning theory, and cognitivism is unconcerned with intra-psychic dynamisms as in psychodynamic theory. According to cognitivism, the central perspective is human thought and its process. Just as a computer thinks, remembers, problem solves, so do humans. Descartes said 'I think therefore I am' and argued that only people thinking through situations can have a sense of personal identity. There has been much critique of this perspective and it is argued by cognitive theorists that a person's life can be planned like a computer; however, it can be counter-argued that emotions get in the way and all too often can ruin the life plan! For instance, people are not usually emotionally moved by things they see or experience literally, but more by the view, or interpretation, they take of what they see or experience.

In terms of child development Piaget (1896–1980) was an extraordinary researcher who has influenced thinking in terms of cognitive development.

Link to Chapter 7 for further discussion on Piaget's stage theory of development.

Humanism

Known as the 'third force' in psychology developed in the United States in the 1950s, the Humanistic approach is an alternate to psychodynamic and learning theory. Humanistic psychologists neither hold the Freudian view that people are driven by forces, or the behaviourists' view that they are manipulated by environment. Humanism argues that people learn from individual experiences, their personal view of events, and from life histories of other people and conclude that this provides more understanding about the meaning of life experience. Humanistic psychologists argue that people are active creatures, essentially good, and capable of choice. There were two main contributors: Carl Rogers (1961) and Abraham Maslow (1970); both argued that human health, growth and positive self-concept come from individual natural tendencies. Maslow developed a humanisitic psychology of motivation; he argues that the individual has a need for self-actualization, is personally responsible, free willed and will strive towards personal growth and fulfilment (Hewstone *et al.* 2006). In Maslow's hierarchy, basic needs must first be gratiated then the individual can move on through other needs to reach a peak in performance (see Figure 6.1).

The four foundational perspectives have all been subject to criticism, as well as found to be fundamental in our learning of psychology, but other theories exist today that make a valuable contribution to our understanding of psychology. This chapter will consider briefly some alternative perspectives to give the reader a taste for further exploration.

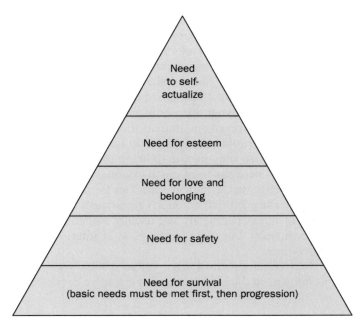

Figure 6.1 Hierarchy of needs
Source: Based on Maslow (1970)

Psycho-biology

This approach seeks to explain human functioning in terms of underlying physical structures and biochemical processes; it seeks to explain behaviour in terms of its physiology, its development, its evolution and its function (Kalat 1995). Psycho-biologists argue that causes of behaviour come from within the nervous system and are pre-wired, affected by hormones and biochemical brain structures. The trigger for action comes from chemical and electrical activities taking place within and between nerve cells. Psycho-biologists question how heredity influences behaviour; they argue that behaviour is a product of our evolutionary history. However, did history leave us with genes that make us think and act in a certain way, or do our genes allow for adaptability to the environment so that our thinking and behaviour is a product of our upbringing? This is a question that has been asked in much research over time including studies on twins and adopted children (Sternberg *et al.* 2003).

Social cultural theory

This theory was brought about by contemporary social scientists in the analysis of the social origins of mental processes. In this view, mental functioning in the individual can be understood only by examining the social and cultural processes e.g. the family, environment, culture and so on, from which the individual derives. Humans are nurtured in a social world and within differing cultural diversities. Consequently, this must have an impact on the behaviour of the individual. Vygotsky (1961) argued that development and mental functioning occurs through external factors. Vygotsky theorized that individuals have a Zone of Proximal Development (ZPD) in which development occurs, from a human being totally dependent and supported in learning a new skill ('scaffolding') to being facilitated and guided (guided participation) to becoming independent (see Figure 7.1 on page 91).

Link to Chapter 7 for further discussion on Vygotsky.

Social constructionism

Social constructionism is a non-scientific approach to psychology along with humanism. This approach is based on the assumption that our knowledge of ourselves and of others is socially constructed, consequently there is no objective reality. In other words, social construction is about understanding the behaviour of human beings based on what the current thinking is, so what are called facts are simply versions of events, which in modern-day society are acceptable. Social constructionism argues that human beings are always a product of their cultural and personal history and of their immediate social contexts. This approach directs study away from individual behaviour, towards a study of relationships examining human practices and discourses (experiences and language). Social constructionism argues that knowledge is inherently dependent on communication of shared meaning and therefore will always be ruled by principles of conduct. Social constructionism informs us of how to behave in a given group.

The approaches discussed briefly above are not exhaustive; they have been chosen to provide readers with an awareness of the topic of psychology, and hopefully encourage them towards further reading. Theories often contradict, but sometimes complement each other. However, they all pursue the accumulation of knowledge. In psychology there are many theories based on several schools of thought or approaches. In order to relate the perspectives discussed above to the practice of the healthcare professional, this chapter will follow with a case study that considers a situation from some of these perspectives. Hopefully this will aid the reader in terms of the application of psychology to practice.

Case study

Shaun is a 19-year-old first-year student at university. He is doing well in his studies and enjoying his programme so far. However, he finds it extremely difficult to participate in seminars and workshops and experiences extreme stress prior to these sessions and suffers physiological symptoms of nausea, sweating, stammering, dry mouth and cough. In these situations Shaun feels faint and gets angry with himself, as he has no control over these experiences.

While reading this summary you may well have come to the conclusion that Shaun suffers from anxiety; you are correct.

Link to Chapter 8 for more on anxiety.

 Stop and think – What would the differing approaches to psychology above make of Shaun's experience?

Psychodynamic approach

From a psychoanalytic view, Shaun's anxiety may well be a symptom of problems dating back to his relationship with his parents when growing up. He may have had difficulty in speaking out in the family home; it may be that one of his parents was very dominant and he found it easier to remain silent. It could be that Shaun experienced conflict at the stage of development in which he was trying to find his own identity when he was trying to establish sexual, political and career identities or was confused about what roles to play. Identity crises can create storm and stress. A psychotherapist could help Shaun to find out and come to terms with his anxiety or repressed problem and help him to alter his responses to the situational factors that make him anxious including 'speaking out in class'.

Learning theory (Behaviourist approach)

Shaun could have experienced in his early life a situation in which he felt extreme anxiety in a classroom: that could be enough to generate anxiety in similar future situations. This is known as a conditioned emotional response or learned behaviour, and arises, according to learning theory, from classical conditioning. Classical conditioning (in a nutshell) occurs when a stimulus (event or situation) triggers anxiety because it has previously been associated with another threatening stimulus and negative response.

Behaviourists would be most concerned with the circumstance in which the anxiety occurs (Antecedent) the behaviour itself and the consequence (ABC) and not concerned with the thoughts and feelings being suffered. This is termed functional analysis of behaviour. It may be that Shaun has previously experienced, for argument's sake a situation in which he gave a presentation and forgot his note cards and felt very embarrassed, which produced anxiety. This situation would have negative consequences for further presentations. This behaviour is bought about by operant conditioning based on the law of effect.

Cognitivist approach

The cognitivist would consider Shaun's situation in terms of his previous experience, like the behaviourist, but would want to know how Shaun interprets the problem and how he has processed the information that causes the anxiety. A cognitivist would consider the interpretation as the basis for changing the way Shaun thinks about the problem that causes the anxiety. If the anxiety was such that it became debilitating, Shaun might be offered cognitive behaviour therapy (CBT).

Humanist approach

The humanist would be interested in Shaun's self-esteem. How does he perceive his abilities? Does Shaun have a perception of himself as a failure when having to 'speak out' in public? The humanist may consider that Shaun would benefit from client-centred therapy and maybe refer him to the student counselling service. This would provide Shaun with the opportunity to talk through his fears and to gain insight into what worries him and why. The intended outcome would be that Shaun gains confidence and feels better about himself and would experience far less anxiety when participating in seminars or workshops and speaking out in class.

Psychology can be considered a difficult subject to understand and the study of it has two sides, one that deals in the absolute scientific reality, learned through experimentation, and the other that appears to be common sense, logical and easily understood, which is socially constructed. One deals in facts and the other deals in meanings that can change over time and in different situations and circumstances. The study of human behaviour has over many years enabled psychologists to understand how certain psychological problems may arise and how they can be managed. In terms of providing health care, the understanding of how people think and why they behave as they do can only be a valuable resource for the healthcare professional.

Psychology has been considered not as essential as physiology and sociology, suggesting that these subject areas are different parts that form a whole. Today, it is generally agreed amongst healthcare professionals that these parts are all equally important and health care is provided with consideration for a holistic approach; the whole is made up of equal parts (Payne and Walker 2000).

Conclusion

Hopefully, this chapter has provided you with a taste of the exciting subject of psychology and a thirst for more. Psychology is a core subject for the healthcare professional, along with sociology and physiology. However, it can be a difficult subject to follow in terms of its relevance to health care. Psychologists like to debate differing ideas; if you study psychology you will join this interesting debate.

 Stop and think – about the differing perspectives. Which do you think makes most sense? Which aligns to your practice more readily? Challenge the basic assumptions and ask your own questions.

The following chapter is focused on developmental psychology; please do read on.

Chapter key points

- Ambulance clinicians require an understanding of psychology in order to care holistically for patients/clients and their families.
- The case study within the chapter clearly explains the value of understanding psychology and linking theory with practice.

References and suggested reading

Atkinson, R.L., Smith, E.D. and Hilgard, E.P. (2003) *Introduction to Psychology*. Belmont, CA: Wadsworth.

Berryman, J., Ockleford, E., Howells, K., Hargreaves, D. and Wildbur, D. (2006) *Psychology and You. An Informal Introduction*, 3rd edn. Oxford: British Psychological Society and Blackwell.

Berryman, J.C., Smyth, P.K., Taylor, A., Lemont, A. and Joiner, R. (2002) *Developmental Psychology and You*. Oxford: British Psychological Society and Blackwell.

Broadbent, D. (1958) *Perception and Communication*. London: Pergamon Press.

Edelmann, R.J. (2000) *Psycho-social Aspects of the Healthcare Process*. Marlow: Pearson Education.

Eysenck, H.J. (2000) *Psychology: A Student's Handbook*. Hove: Psychology Press.

Eysenck, H.J. and Eysenck, M.W. (1981) *Personality and Individual Differences: A Natural Science Approach*. New York: Plenum.

Freud, S. (1975) Inhibitions, symptoms and anxiety, in *The Standard Education of the Complete Psychological works of Sigmund Freud*. London: Hogarth Press, originally published 1926.

Gross, R. (2001) *Psychology: The Science of Mind and Behaviour*. London: Hodder and Stoughton.

Hewstone, M., Fincham, F.D. and Foster, J. (2006) *Psychology*. Oxford: British Psychological Society and Blackwell.

Kalat, J.H. (1995) *Biological Psychology*, 5th edn. Pacific Grove, CA: Brooks/Cole Publishing.

Kohlberg, L., Levine, C. and Hewer, A. (1983) *Moral Stages: A Current Reformulation and a Response to Critics*. New York: Basal.

Maslow A.H. (1970) *Toward a Psychology of Being*, 3rd edn. New York: Van Nostrand.

Ogden, J. (2000) *Health Psychology: A Textbook*, 2nd edn. Buckingham: OU Press.

Palmer, J.A. (2005) *Fifty Modern Thinkers on Education, from Piaget to the Present*. Oxford: Routledge.

Pavlov, I.P. (1927) *Conditioned Reflexes*. London: Oxford University Press.

Payne, S. and Walker, J. (2000) *Psychology for Nurses and the Caring Professions*. Buckingham: OU Press.

Piaget, J. and Enhelder, B. (1967) *The Psychology of the Child*. London: Routledge.

Rogers, C. R. (1961) *On Becoming a Person*. Boston, MA: Howton.

Skinner, B.F. (1974) *About Behaviourism*. London: Jonathon Cape.

Sternberg, R.J., Lautrey, J. and Lubart, T.I. (eds) (2003). *Models of Intelligence: International Perspectives*. Washington, DC: American Psychological Association.

Vygotsky, L. (1961) *Thought and Language*. Boston, MA: MIT Press.

Zimbardo, P., McDermott, M., Jansz, J. and Metaal, N. (1995) *Psychology: A European Text.* London: Harper Collins.

Useful website

Portland State University, Department of Psychology. The Psi Café Link: *www.psy.pdx.edu*

7

Developmental psychology: an introduction
Jackie Whitnell

Topics covered:

- Introduction
- Why is this relevant?
- Theories of development
- Examples of different approaches for the same situation depending on the age and stage of development of the child
- Atypical development
- Conclusion
- Chapter key points
- References, suggested reading and useful websites

Introduction

The lifespan approach is commonly used in developmental psychology – from conception to the elderly. This introductory text will consider developmental psychology from birth to young adulthood. However, I would advise the healthcare professional to take time to read around the important development that occurs at conception and during pregnancy.

Research can be conducted over different time spans, from a few seconds or minutes of observation to months, years or even an entire lifetime, as with longitudinal research. This is seen in developmental psychology and is vital in terms of understanding what occurs at stages and ages of children and young adults. This chapter will first look at the importance of the ambulance clinician having an understanding of child development (developmental psychology). Having taught this subject to student ambulance clinicians, I am often greeted in the first instance with a query as to why they need this knowledge, so I am taking this opportunity of providing the answer to that question before I continue, in the hope that you do not skip this chapter! This chapter will provide you with an awareness of the different approaches to child development and will relate these to your everyday practice of caring for children and their parents/carers. This chapter will consider, albeit briefly, atypical development (learning disabilities), to provide the reader with an overview of the diversity of children's development.

Why is this relevant?

After considering some of the approaches of psychology in the previous chapter, you could ask 'Why is it important for me as an ambulance clinician or healthcare professional to have an understanding of developmental psychology (child development) when caring for children? How will the theory link to my practice?' You will, maybe for a short yet extremely valuable period of time, be caring for children and their family members; in that time your knowledge base around how a child develops could be essential.

 Stop and think – Before reading on, why not jot down why you think it is important for you to have an understanding of child development?

If you have an understanding of normal child development you will be in a better position to:

- understand why children and families behave in the way that they do;
- relate to the child, so he has an appropriate understanding of what you are asking of him and why;
- have an awareness of what to expect in terms of the child's language (according to 'usual' stage of development), which will aid communication in order to obtain accurate information regarding her health needs;
- make a more accurate assessment regarding learning needs, special needs, disability, pain, and so on. Only the child can tell you how he feels (if able to express it); the mother/father can only describe what she/he has seen or heard;
- be able to 'pitch' your communication at the appropriate level for age/stage and understanding;
- observe the child's behaviour and social interaction with her carer. This can be extremely valuable information, especially for situations where non-accidental injury is a possible concern;
- identify inappropriate behaviour for age/stage of development and be able to inform the professional of your worries when handing over the child's care;
- use evidence-based knowledge from differing perspectives of child development when caring for the child;
- have an awareness of children's rights;
- inform Emergency Department staff and other healthcare professionals of

concerns, in order that the child can be followed up appropriately, safeguarding the child at all times;

● be able to complete appropriately, and with knowledge base, the patient report form and if necessary the safeguarding children report form.

Link to chapter 9 for more detail on policy and practice on this topic

How well did you do with your own thoughts?

Do read on to gain a greater understanding of developmental psychology.

Theories of development

Attachment theory

Most of infants' early learning is in social development. There are two main aspects of this early learning that are very important: sociability and attachment. As an ambulance clinician you will observe relationships between child and carer and you may well try to administer care to the infant/child. You may experience a crying child, clinging to its carer and trying to get away from your care; this could be due to what is termed *stranger awareness*. Stranger awareness usually occurs around the age of 8 months when the child develops object permanence.

Link to Piaget's sensori-motor stage of development discussed further on in this chapter.

At this stage the child knows the difference between a familiar face and that of a stranger; it highlights that the child's cognitive development (thinking) and social development is taking place. At approximately 8–12 months most children will try to cling on to their carer. When you try to remove them for a short while they will cry out, but will stop crying and smile almost as soon as you pass them back to their familiar carer. There has been much research on attachment theory and you might like to read Mary Ainsworth (1979) on infant–mother attachment, which discusses what she terms 'strange situations'.

John Bowlby (1979) argued that although the main attachment of an infant is usually to its mother, strong bonds occur to significant others with whom the infant has regular contact. If as an ambulance clinician it is essential you administer treatment to a child it would always be better (if possible) for you to have the person with the child to whom the child is attached; this may make your administering care a lot easier. There are three stages in early development of attachment to others: the asocial

Biography

John Bowlby (1907–90), child psychiatrist and psychoanalyst, was the first to describe the importance of attachment in human development. His interest in the study of animal behaviour led to his theory that human children, like young animals, have a need for a figure that provides a source of safety, comfort and protection.

stage; the stage of indiscriminate attachment; and the stage of specific attachments. According to Freud's psychodynamic approach, babies are initially attached to their mother because she provides nourishment. However, there is no simple link between food and attachment behaviour, as was found in research by Harlow *et al.* (1971). Harlow observed that monkeys *attached* to a cloth mother who provided nourishment as opposed to the same nourishment provided by a mother made of wire. It was the blanket that the monkeys attached to, not the food.

According to Bowlby, infants have an innate tendency to form strong bonds with a particular individual, and there is a critical period which ends by the age of 3 years. According to Bowlby, in the first three years of life bonding must occur. In contrast, Ainsworth (1979) found that the relationship between the mother and baby develops over time, rather than being fixed shortly after birth. Evidence from the 'strange situations' test indicates that there are three main types of attachment of infants to their mother: secure attachment; anxious and resistant attachment; and anxious and avoidant attachment. You will note that not all attachment is positive! According to this care-giving hypothesis, the sensitivity of the mother (or significant other) is of great importance in determining the type of attachment. However, this hypothesis does not take into account the part played by the infant, and infers the mother's sensitivity and responsiveness.

In reality, not all infants and children are parented sensitively or responsively. As an ambulance clinician you will observe many different/diverse parenting skills. Deprivation can lead to long-term difficulties when it occurs due to problems with social relationships, more than from ill-health. Bowlby (1979) argued that adverse effects of maternal deprivation are normally irreversible. Cultural differences in parenting practices reflect differences in terms of adults' cultural expectations and values. Parental acceptance and rejection can vary in different cultures but, in the main, rejection is generally associated with poor outcome in the children, e.g. low self-esteem, delinquency and possibly aggression. This can also have a knock-on effect on educational attainment at school. Having acknowledged the different types of attachment, it is incumbent upon me to say that most infants in most cultures have a secure attachment and as an ambulance clinician you will most often see positive attachment between child and carer throughout your daily practice.

Stop and think – Consider the relationships between parent and child that you have cared for. Have they always been warm and caring? As an ambulance clinician you are in a prime position to notice the interaction between the child

and carer and it is important that you report anything that is untoward or
inappropriate when you hand over the care of the child.

Psychoanalytical and learning theory

Grand theories are comprehensive theories that have inspired and directed thinking
about development over decades, but no longer seem as adequate as they once did.
However, they remain influential.

During the first half of the twentieth century, two opposing grand theories dominated the child development 'scene':

1   Psychoanalytic theory (Psycho-sexual=Freud; Psycho-social=Erikson)
2   Learning theory (Behaviourism) – Thorndike/Watson/Skinner/Pavlov

These began as psychological theories and later applied to human developmental
psychology theories more broadly. A fundamental assumption of psychoanalytic theory is that development over the lifespan is determined during early childhood.

Psycho-sexual theory

Freud argued that we are born with two instinctive urges (libido and death wish),
which provide psychic energy. This theory holds that irrational, unconscious forces,
many of them from childhood, underlie human behaviour.

Biography

Sigmund Freud (1856–1939) was not a psychologist. He was a Viennese physician,
referred to as 'the father of psychoanalysis'. He was interested in the role of
unconscious mental processes and inner forces (id, ego, and super ego) that he
considered influenced people's behaviour.

Urges are gratified by three parts of personality, through stages of development which
reflect erogenous zones:

Box 7.1 Freud's stages of psychosexual development

Stage	Average age	Development
Oral	0–18mths	Eating and sucking provides satisfaction
Anal	18–36mths	Anal area is interesting and satisfying
Phallic	3–5yrs	Satisfaction from the genitals
Latency	6 yrs–puberty	Boys and girls spend little time together
Genital	Onset of puberty	Main pleasure from genitals

These underlying forces (id, ego and super ego) and urges influence people's thinking
and behaviour in the smallest decisions and in crucial life changes.

Drives and motive provide foundation for universal stages of development in human experience. A critique of this theory of development is that it is one-sided, the emphasis being on sexuality as the dynamic factor in development. Theorists from other approaches acknowledge Freud's thinking even though it is considered empirically weak (Hewstone *et al.* 2005). An important example of radical reformulation of psycho-sexual development theory is Erikson's psycho-social theory.

Biography

Erik Erikson (1902–94) was a Jewish German developmental psychologist who coined the phrase 'identity crisis'.

He was one of Freud's followers who accepted some of Freud's theory and expanded it to take into account people's lifestyle and culture. He argued that child rearing can only be understood by making reference to the competencies valued and needed by the individual's society.

Psycho-social theory

Erikson acknowledged the importance of the unconscious; he agreed that unresolved childhood conflicts at certain stages affect adulthood, but expanded and modified Freud's ideas. Erikson proposed eight developmental stages, each characterized by a particular challenge or developmental crisis, which is central to that stage of life. He placed emphasis on a person's relationship to his family and culture; not just sexual urges.

Link to Chapter 11 to explore areas of our lives that influence our personal and social development

---

Erikson argued that resolutions to conflicts depend on interactions with others in the social world. Each stage of development has a conflict and resolution. According to Erikson, in order to develop positively one has to resolve each stage of conflict to move on to the next stage of development. It may be problematic if a person is static in a stage of conflict and that may predispose to difficulties in a person's future development. His stages are as follows:

1 Trust vs mistrust (birth to 1 year)

   Babies learn either to trust that others will care for their basic needs, including nourishment, warmth, cleanliness and physical contact, or will lack confidence in the care given by others.

2 Autonomy vs shame and doubt (1 year to 3 years)

   Children learn either to be self-sufficient in many activities, including toileting, feeding, walking, exploring and talking, or they may doubt their own abilities.

3   Initiative vs guilt (3 years to 6 years)

Children want to undertake many adult-like activities, sometimes overstepping the limits set by parents. That can lead to the child feeling guilty, thus resulting in poor self-esteem.

Stop and think – As an ambulance clinician you will identify Stages 2 and 3 in terms of children who have attempted something that may well have been out of their range of development, which results in an accident.

4   Industry vs inferiority (6 years to 11 years)

Children busily learn to be competent and productive in mastering new skills or they may feel inferior and unable to do anything well.

Stop and think – Stage 4 is a stage of development that can predispose to child and adolescent mental health issues. A child may experience the feeling of being worthless, unable to achieve, leading to the potential for depression.

5   Identity vs role confusion (Adolescence)

Adolescents try to figure out 'Who am I?'

They establish sexual, political and career identities or may be confused about what roles to play. Identity crises can create storm and stress for the young person. Sociological theory suggests that changes within social roles cause conflicts, e.g. girlfriend and daughter, schoolgirl and work experience. In addition, mass media and peers can cause conflicting values for this age. It can be a very difficult time for the young person going through this stage of development (Muuss 1996; Kroger 2000; Berryman *et al.* 2006).

6   Intimacy vs isolation – (young adult)

Young people are working on establishing intimate ties to others. However, if they have experienced earlier attachment problems some young adults cannot form close relationships and remain isolated.

7   Generativity vs stagnation – (middle adulthood)

This stage involves giving to and guiding the next generation through child rearing, caring for others or reproduction. If a person cannot achieve this they may feel an absence of meaningful accomplishment.

8   Ego integrity vs despair (the elderly person)

This is the final stage where people reflect on the kind of person they have been and become. Integrity comes from feeling that life is worth living. However, older people who are not happy with their life fear death (Berger 2003; Berk 2003).

Learning theory is considered a more acceptable theory of child development and holds with the view that all development involves a change in an individual. Behaviourism and the law of learning theory are based on the premise that learning can be explained by the forming of associations. Learning involves a *stimulus* (action which elicits a response) and *response* (instinct or learned action taken upon the stimulus) through *conditioning*. There are two types of conditioning associated with behaviourism:

Classical conditioning

This conditioning was demonstrated by Ivan Pavlov (1849–1936) (Pavlov 1927). His research on dogs demonstrated the salivary conditioned reflex in dogs (learning by association), for which he is widely known today. Pavlov was studying dogs' reflex salivation in response to food, and was surprised to observe that the dogs salivated on some occasions when they had no food. He found food (which always induced salivation) became an 'unconditional stimulus' (UCS) and the response of salivation was the 'unconditional response' (UCR). In his experiments Pavlov always sounded a bell every time the dogs were fed, just before they were given any food. After this had been repeated many times, he sounded the bell without giving any food, yet the dogs still salivated = learned behaviour.

Biography

John Watson (1876–1958) was opposed to Freud and Erikson's ideas on development and offered a new type of psychology. He argued that psychologists should study only what they could see and measure, not the unconscious. According to Watson, anything could be learned; in the right environment he could train anyone to be anything regardless of talents, tendencies, abilities, vocations and cultures. He argued that the study of actual behaviour is objective and far less difficult than the study of unconscious motives and drives. Watson extended Pavlov's research and showed that classical conditioning occurred also in humans.

Watson's research could be considered simplistic and we cannot explain all learning by stimulus–response associations. However, there are many situations that can illicit a response that is pleasurable and/or uncomfortable, e.g. places, music, smells, photos or pictures. Consequently, one could argue that there is a lot to be said for classical conditioning.

Operant conditioning

This conditioning occurs when behaviour produces a consequence.

Edward Lee Thorndike (1874–1949) and Burrhus Frederic Skinner (biologist then psychologist) (1904–90) agreed with Watson and Pavlov, but found that operant conditioning plays a greater role in human behaviour. Operant conditioning occurs when an association is formed between a response and its consequences. The proposed law of effect found that reward will strengthen the connection between the response that preceded it and any stimuli present when it is delivered. The principle is that the consequence (effect) of behaviour will determine how likely it is to recur; for example, if the consequence of behaviour is useful/pleasure/relieving (a positive reinforcement, such as medication), a child will take the medication again, when instructed, to achieve that same consequence (effect). Conditioning is used quite widely in behaviour management of children and in managing people who suffer with phobias (Hewstone *et al.* 2005).

 Stop and think – If a child experiences an asthmatic attack and is given a nebulizer, which makes the child feel much better and less scared, the child will be happy to use it again. Reinforcement and reward is very useful when managing a child who is scared; learning theory used in practice can be very useful. The child has learned that the response to her difficult breathing comes from the positive reward of the nebulizer = operant conditioning.

Learning theory or behaviourism is practical and avoids references to the unconscious which cannot be observed, measured or proved to exist. Behaviour is observable and so are many of its causes. However, conditioning does not adequately explain where new behaviour comes from; social learning theory may help to explain this.

Social learning theory

This approach argues that not all learning has occurred from the child's experience of direct classical or operant conditioning (behaviourism). Children learn to behave in ways that are rewarding and avoid ways that are punished by others (Carpendale and Lewis 2006). Social learning theory, a more recent approach, accepts that children learn from reinforcement and punishment but also suggests that they learn by observing, imitating and modelling on others. Modelling occurs when the observer is uncertain or inexperienced and models on a more senior, admired, powerful role model (Bandura 1977).

 Stop and think – If a child needs medication or a plaster for example, you could consider this theory to aid administration. You could use modelling in terms of pretending to give the medication to the child's doll or teddy or put the plaster/ bandage on the doll or teddy. Upon seeing this situation and with the intention of modelling the behaviour the child may have more confidence in your doing it to him.

Cognitive theory

Two grand theories have been discussed: that of psychodynamic theory and behaviourism. In the middle of the twentieth century these theories were joined by a third grand theory: cognitive theory. This is well known, as is the theorist: Piaget.

Biography

Jean Piaget (1896–1980) was a biologist and zoologist from Switzerland. Piaget's basic idea argued that it is more useful to understand how a child stores and uses information than how much knowledge and intellect a child has.
Study of three areas:
- how the senses take in information about things around us;
- how the brain processes and stores information;
- how the subsequent behaviour changes as a result of stored information = cognitive theory of development.

Piaget was a very influential and extraordinary intellectual leader/researcher who fashioned the framework of cognitive theory. Piaget argued that the focus of development is on structure and development of the individual thought processes and how they affect the person's understanding of the world. He also argued that development does not occur through what has been forgotten (Freud, Erikson) or what has been learned (Pavlov, Skinner), but from what and how children think. Understanding how children think reveals how they interpret their experience and explains how they construct their understanding of the world.

Piaget found that children develop in stages. There are four stages of development, which are age-related, in which changes take place, the first stage being the most dramatic.

Let us look at these stages in turn:

1 Sensori motor
2 Pre-operational
3 Concrete operational
4 Formal operational

1 Sensori motor stage, 0–2 years

The most dynamic stage of a child's life. Most changes take place, from simple physical reflexes through to beginning to symbolize.

Initially an infant's interactions are basic and reflexive but after a very short time the baby will learn to use some muscles and limbs for movement, and will begin to understand some information received through her senses.

 Stop and think – What are the senses? Jot them down and consider why they are important.

The first ideas babies develop are about how to deal with their world; these are called 'action schemas' (construct representations of events, people and relationships from the real physical world). Babies are totally egocentric; they are unable to take anyone else's needs or interests into account. They start to develop fine and gross motor skills, become social beings and develop language (see Sheridan *et al.* 2007 for detail on the development of these skills in weeks, months and early years, and Carpendale and Lewis 2006). Infants learn about objects and what they can be made to do. Some intellectual behaviour is occurring, for example they will hold a rattle and shake it, then throw it and watch what happens to it. Objects start to have meaning and babies/infants begin to do more with them. This is the time when object permanence occurs. Piaget found that object permanence occurs at around 6–8 months of age. However, Baillargeon *et al.* (1985) found that children have object permanence at a much earlier age – around 4–5 months. Object permanence is when a child is aware cognitively that an object exists, even though it is not in sight. For example, if a toy is placed in front of a child for view and then a cover is placed over the toy to conceal it, the child will think the toy has gone, unless the child has cognitively developed object permanence. If the child has developed this concept she will lift the cloth covering the object and expect to see the toy.

2 Pre-operational stage, 2–7 years

Operations at this stage will require combining schemas in an orderly, sensible, logical way, although at this stage they will be somewhat limited. The child's vocabulary and imagination is expanding at 2 years, seen in the use of words in play such as house, mummy, car, bird, dog, cat and so on, and they may not be heard clearly. At the beginning of this stage, the child understands much of what is being said to him but can find it difficult to express himself; this brings about frustration. At around 3 years onwards you may well hear two- to three-word sentences: Daddy gone work; Mummy feed dog. From around 4 years onwards fuller sentence structure occurs. There is again a great deal of difference in development from 2 years to 7 years (see Sheridan *et al.* 2007 for further information).

Within this stage the child is beginning to use:

- Symbolism – children's thought processes are developing; they are starting to make sense of their world and make use of symbolization – symbols that stand for something, or to symbolize something else, for instance a thumbs up symbol for agreement/happy.

 Stop and think – Symbols such as thumbs up can be extremely valuable non-verbal communication and inform you as the healthcare professional as to how the child is feeling.

Link to Chapter 3 for additional means of general communication

- Egocentrism – child generally sees things from her own point of view. The child assumes that everyone will experience what she is experiencing with the same meaning and that everyone will feel as she does.

Stop and think – You could use a doll or teddy to aid assistance. Not all children at this stage are egotistical; if the task is simple he may be able to see it from others' perspectives depending on where he is in the stage of development.

- Animism – child holds with the belief that everything that exists has some kind of consciousness. For example, if the car won't start, the car is tired; if the child is hurt in a collision with chair, she will blame the 'naughty chair'.

- Moral realism (later in the stage) – the child thinks that her way of thinking about what is right and wrong will be shared by everyone else. She will focus on one aspect of a situation at a time. She will have respect for rules and they have to be obeyed; cannot take motives into account. She does not grasp the finality of death and feels she is to blame for sudden deaths.

Stop and think – At this stage the use of moral realism may well help you to administer treatment. If you explain that the treatment is essential for the child's well-being the child may well respect your decision making.

3 Concrete operational stage, 7–11 years

At this stage you will experience a child with more rational and adult-like thinking. There is more logical reasoning and grasp of the idea that illness and death have biological causes. At this stage the child recognizes her own mortality. This is an easier stage in the child's life, where you can explain what has happened and what you are going to do about it.

Children can think logically, if they can manipulate the actual object that they are thinking about. At this stage the child learns that objects are not always what they appear, for example conservation, number, volume, length, mass. For example, if you put equal amounts of water into two different cups, one tall and thin and one short and wide, the child will probably know that there is the same amount of water in both cups. However, if the child has not cognitively developed 'conservation' he may believe that the tall, thin cup holds more water (because it looks more to the eye), even though you have shown him the same amount of water being poured into the two cups (Keenan 2002).

4 Formal operational stage, 11–16 years

At this stage children can manipulate their thoughts, and do not need the real object at hand.

Around puberty, the ways in which children think change again. They work things out in their heads, without seeing the object; they think more abstractly, consider a range of societal issues and can take others' reasons for behaviour into account. However, not all young people, nor indeed some adults, can do this, as they may not have developed to this stage cognitively. According to Piaget, at this stage young adults can understand the link between biology and psychology, between feelings and symptoms. They tend to be better able to comprehend more immediate and short-term risks, but are less able to understand the longer term consequences of their behaviours (Davenport 2002; Keenan 2002; Berger 2003; Berk 2003).

Box 7.2 Domains of development

Biological	*Cognitive*	*Psycho-social*
Genes	Perception	Temperament
Hormones	Memory	Family
Information processing	Imagination	Culture
Motor skills	Learning	Values
Fine motor skills	Thinking	Beliefs
	Decision making	School
	Hearing and speech	Socialization and play
		Significant others

Box 7.2 highlights the areas of development according to the main domains: bio-social, cognitive and psycho-social.

Stop and think – Can you jot down from memory what is expected in terms of physical gross and fine motor skills according to ages and stages of child development, from birth to 5 years? It would be valuable for the ambulance clinician and other health professionals that come into contact with children to have an understanding of basic 'normal' development milestones to aid assessment of children. A useful small text by Sheridan *et al.* (2007) is *Birth to Five Years: Child Developmental Progress*. This text breaks down detailed stages of development.

Piaget was criticized by social constructivists for his underestimation of the role of social and cultural factors in knowledge development, hence the emergence of the socio-cultural theory of development.

Socio-cultural theory

The socio-cultural theory is relatively new when compared with the grand theories of development; it is considered emergent and brings together information from many disciplines. Vygotsky (1962) sought to explain individual knowledge, development and competencies in terms of the guidance, support and structure provided by society.

He argued that development results in a dynamic interaction between child or learner and people, surroundings and culture (normally parents, teachers, peers) that provides instruction and support to the child in order that she can acquire knowledge and capabilities. This theory considers the importance of social factors; children are apprentices in thinking. The concepts of 'scaffolding' and 'guided participation' in acts of everyday life are important for children to draw on. This is acquired through the child learning from experienced members of a social group or people the child considers to be a role model. Children naturally absorb cultural expectations as a part of learning, and development occurs when a child is guided by a more senior, admired role model. Vygotsky developed the concept of the Zone of Proximal Development (ZPD), seen in Figure 7.1 below.

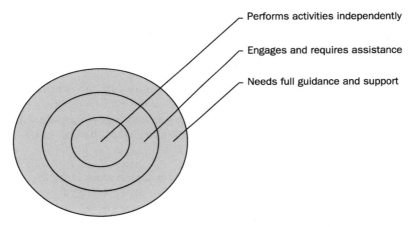

Performs activities independently

Engages and requires assistance

Needs full guidance and support

Figure 7.1 Based on Vygotsky's Zone of Proximal Development

Figure 7.1 highlights the process a child goes through, in terms of learning. The child moves through the learning process from the outer zone (being totally dependent and supported) through the middle zone (being facilitated) to the inner zone where the child becomes fully independent.

Vygotsky (1962) also emphasized the importance of language as a learning tool for children and language being valuable in terms of communicating feelings. He argued that inner speech is a form of language spoken to oneself, for instance in an examination a student could use inner speech to talk through the answer to a question before writing.

This part of the chapter has provided the reader with an understanding of children's development. It will be apparent that there are not only different theoretical approaches to child development but also different stages at which the child develops. Below are examples of two situations that you can relate to in children of different ages, in terms of practical care.

> **Biography**
>
> **Lev Vygotsky** (1896–1934) was one of the most important Russian psychologists of the twentieth century.
>
> Famous for research into development and structure of human consciousness, and theory of signs, which explains the way children internalize language in the course of their social and cultural development.
>
> 'Culture is the product of social life and human social activity. That is why just by raising the question of the cultural development of behaviour we are directly introducing the social plane of development.'

Examples of different approaches for the same situation depending on the age and stage of development of the child

When caring for children at different ages and stages of development there will be differing ways to approach the child in order that you can care appropriately, for example:

Below highlights the different ways in which you may care for a child with breathing difficulties who is requiring an oxygen mask and makes the link to the developmental theory behind the management.

- At 6–9 months of age you may show the child what the mask looks like on a teddy or doll before attempting to use it on the child in order that he allows you to care for him. A child will copy/mimic behaviour if it appears to be 'OK'. This aligns to modelling behaviour within social learning theory (Bandura).
- At 5 years of age the child grasps and understands that illness has a biological cause and she needs help, but may be assertive and refuse. It is necessary to explain to a child of this age the importance of the mask and the reasoning behind its use in quite simple terms. This situation in terms of development aligns with Piaget and cognitive theory; this child is likely to be at the pre-operational stage of development. This child's efforts to act independently can lead to pride or failure according to Erikson. This age child is at the initiative vs guilt stage within psychosocial theory.
- At 12 years of age this child would be within the formal operational stage of development according to Piaget. His thinking is more refined and he can comprehend more immediate risks and will accept help and understand why he requires the oxygen via a mask.

Below highlights the different ways in which you may care for a child who is experiencing pain at different ages and considers theories of development.

- At 2 years of age the child may cry out, 'it hurts' or 'sore' and possibly hold the painful area whilst crying. This age child is unlikely to communicate verbally. You will need this child's comforter to help settle her if possible. This child will be 'stranger aware' and cling to carer; you may need to administer the treatment to the child in the carer's arms. This child is at the end of the sensori-motor stage according to Piaget, and has made attachment to the carer according to Bowlby.

- At 5 years this age child will show you where the pain is and point to a pain chart of images/faces to gauge the amount of pain she is experiencing. She may show you on the teddy or doll where the pain is. According to Piaget's pre-operational stage of development this child may have a cognitive understanding of moral realism.

- At 11 years the child will be able to tell you on a scale of 1–10 how bad it is. Pain experience can be mediated by socio-cultural factors (e.g. verbal/nonverbal cues given off by the carer). However, it is imperative that as an ambulance clinician you always believe what the child says until the child is investigated. If the child has been rewarded for his behaviour previously he may have learned to behave in this way. The theory behind this idea comes from positive reinforcement/operant conditioning. This child may have experienced pain in the past and had a positive outcome from medication in which case the child may be happy to accept pain relief; this situation links with the theory on classical conditioning.

Atypical development

As an ambulance clinician or healthcare professional, you are likely to care for and transport children with special needs or learning disability. As this is an introductory text this chapter includes limited discussion of emotional, behavioural and social problems and learning disabilities that children can experience. Therefore, this section will include an example of disorders that will lead to atypical development such as attention deficit hyperactive disorder (ADHD), autistic spectrum disorder and children who have Down's syndrome. It is important that you have an understanding of the diversity of children's development in order that you care for them appropriately. In the first instance, it is incumbent upon me to say that children with learning disabilities are in fact children first, with needs and rights similar to those of any other child. They will have other special needs but the understanding and management of those needs (albeit in some instances challenging) will affect the outcome. There are many difficulties that all children can face and it is important that healthcare professionals are aware of the potential additional risk of harm for children with learning disabilities and the need to protect them and consider their rights along with all other children (HM Government 1991). I hope that this section will offer *food for thought* and that you will be interested enough to search for further information on children with atypical development by way of self-directed learning.

How do healthcare professionals/psychologists/psychiatrists view developmental psychopathology? The study of developmental psychopathology is thought of as a relationship between psychology and the study of childhood disorders. A range of functions will be taken into account when assessing a child's development e.g. biological, genetic, socio-cultural and cognitive. Psychologists generally assume a continuum of behaviour, with the child's behaviour showing somewhere along it (Comer

2004). There are a number of factors that may contribute to, or result in, learning disabilities. The preconceptual, prenatal, perinatal and postnatal periods are distinct and differing times, before and during pregnancy and after birth, when learning disabilities can occur, as these are the times when possible causative factors operate. These factors are:

- heredity (the gene is a discrete segment of the chromosome and the basic unit for the transition of heredity instructions e.g. hair and eye colour traits. The chromosome is the carrier of genes. An example of chromosomal abnormality is Down's Syndrome; see atypical development for further details) and;
- environment during and after pregnancy: toxic agents, birth trauma, oxygen starvation, nutrition (Gates 2007).

How do professionals diagnose children with atypical development? How do they know when normal behaviour ends and developmental psychopathology begins? Children differ considerably in their rate of development, and it makes sense to continue to think in terms of the stages of development that most children go through at around the same ages. However, these stages are less relevant to those children who, for a number of reasons, are not developing as per the *normal* age and stage.

There are many ways of determining whether someone has a learning disability; however, no one criterion will provide a definitive answer. Over time, psychiatrists and researchers have highlighted the confusion of diagnosis and the use of different tools (Morton 2004). Defining learning disability is difficult as it means different things to different people. Generally it is agreed that learning disability comprises of sub-average intellectual functioning that coexists with below-average social functioning that manifests before the age of 18 years (Gates 2007).

Children with learning disability fall into three main areas and can be assessed using differing diagnostic tools:

1 Intellectual ability (Intelligent Quotient = IQ); DSM IV (2000); Child Behaviour Checklist (CBCL) (2003).
2 Legislative definitions: Mental Health Act (1983/2007).
3 Social competence criterion.

Children who have learning disability will have an IQ which is below the average IQ of 100. IQ is useful only up to the age of 18 years. IQ within the population is evenly distributed therefore it is possible to measure how far an individual is from what is considered 'normal'. Using this system, a child who has an IQ of less than 70 is said to have a learning disability (scores more than 2 standard deviations (SD) from the average of 100; score of 15 = 1 SD).

- 70–84 = borderline of intellectual functioning
- 50–69 = mild learning disability (25–30 people in UK per 1000 population)
- 35–49 = moderate learning disability

- 20–34 = severe mental retardation (3–4 people in UK per 1000 population)
- <20 = profound mental retardation (people with complex additional disabilities e.g. sensory, physical or behavioural (Gates 2007).

In legislative terms, children who have physical and sensory impairment, for example who are blind or deaf or suffer from cerebral palsy, are considered to have a learning disability (Mental Health Act 2007).

Children with emotional and behavioural problems, including autistic spectrum disorders (including Asperger's disorder) and Attention Deficit Hyperactivity Disorder (ADHD), are likely to have impaired social functioning and may be assessed using the social competence criterion (Wilmshurst 2004).

An example of a diagnostic tool is shown in Box 7.3.

Box 7.3 Diagnostic Statistical Manual of Mental Disorders (DSM IV)

DSM IV uses categories to classify behaviour, signs and symptoms logged to enable diagnosis.

DSM IV is not concerned with classification, more with the behaviour expressed; suggesting this helps to remove negative stigma of labelling which only leads to derogation and uninformed understanding.

Critique DSM IV considers developmental issues but does not consider changes in children over time. Disorders can occur as a function of age and change at different ages. E.g. Attention Deficit Hyperactive Disorder = in young child; more hyperactivity than in older child.

(American Psychiatric Association 2000)

Diagnostic tools

Another useful diagnostic tool is shown in Box 7.4.

Box 7.4 Child Behaviour Checklist (CBCL)

CBCL is dimensional and provides information about the way and how much the individual shows disturbance. Deviation is viewed as continuous from normal (continuum). It allows for changing behaviour. CBCL looks at internal and external scales. Internal disorders include anxiety and depression; external are outward (ADHD) 'acting out' a form of distress including aggression and delinquency.

Children can show both, e.g. be sulky and aggressive at the same time.

Critique Does not include some major disorders, e.g. autism, eating disorders, which DSM IV includes.

(Achenbach 2003)

It can often be difficult to confirm diagnosis of behaviour, as co-morbidity (where two different conditions are present in one child) can occur (Wood *et al.* 2006). For some children with learning disabilities, a precise diagnosis is not possible and a more comprehensive, multi-agency assessment of the child's needs is required. This is obtained using the *Framework for the Assessment of Children in Need and Their Families* (DoH 2000). This assessment includes the parent's needs for support with caring for the child.

This section will consider a small sample of some significant childhood disorders that children experience which will bring into being learning disabilities of one form or another; during your working practice it is very likely you will care for children with a developmental disorder.

Attention Deficit Hyperactive Disorder (ADHD)

Signs and symptoms
- Unable to sit still for any length of time (pattern of restlessness/overactivity)
- Loses things
- Cannot concentrate on tasks, even fun tasks
- Easily distracted
- Doesn't appear to listen (inattentive)
- Much energy, fidgets, runs, climbs, talks incessantly
- Shows antisocial behaviour (impulsive)
- Interrupts conversation

(American Psychiatric Association 2000)

ADHD is an externalizing form of maladjustment. The name of this disorder highlights the issues that arise. It involves the ongoing presence of inattention and hyperactivity with impulsiveness, all of which is beyond the norm and is more frequent and severe. In true ADHD, symptoms are evident in children less than 7 years of age and the behaviour occurs at school and at home (APA 2000). This disorder affects 3 to 5 per cent of the population with a 4:1 male to female ratio, 50 to 80 per cent still into adulthood (Wenar and Kerig 2000; Royal College of Psychiatrists 2001; Morton 2004).

It is difficult to diagnose this in toddlers, as at this age you would expect inattention, but it can be detected if extreme, frequent and chronic. It is easier to detect in middle childhood, as one would expect a child to have more control in their activities, be socially competent and be able to concentrate for a period of time. These children can show antisocial behaviour in adolescence and young adulthood, consequently this disorder may go hand in hand with conduct disorder (co-morbidity). Conduct disorder is defined as 'a repetitive and persistent pattern of behaviour in which the basic rights of others or major age-appropriate societal norms or rules are violated' (APA 2000). Indeed, co-occurrence of conduct disorder and ADHD and their symptoms is so strong that researchers have questioned whether they are separate disorders (Morton 2004).

Autism lies at the extreme end of the autistic spectrum and is characterized by a triad of social communication difficulties. Vygotsky (1962) stated that language, thoughts and social interaction are inextricably linked around the age of 2 years.

Autistic Spectrum Disorders (Pervasive developmental disorders – PDD) (DSM 1V)
Autism Signs and symptoms • Deficits in sociability and empathy • Deficits in communicative language • Deficits in cognitive flexibility • Delay with speech development • Restricted, repetitive and stereotyped patterns of behaviour, interests and activities • Detectable before the age of 3 years • 70 per cent children have < 70 IQ Asperger's syndrome Signs and symptoms • Poor social skills, lack of insight • Behavioural inflexibility, narrow range of interests • IQ > 70 (Note: these children have an IQ that is greater than the criteria for learning disability and indeed can have strengths in verbal areas; Wilmshurst 2004) • No delay with speech; often well developed vocabulary basis but deficit in communication at a social level • Visual motor clumsiness with typical stiff gait and posture Pervasive Developmental Disorder (PDD) not otherwise specified • Applies to less severely affected children who do not meet the criteria for either Autism or Asperger's syndrome. <div align="right">(American Psychiatric Association 2000)</div>

Consequently, this disorder may not be noticed in infancy. These children have impairment in communication and socialization, and restricted and repetitive interests, movements and activities. The prevalence of autistic spectrum disorder has risen between 1992 and 2001, so research focuses on trying to find out why, and what causes it. The factors suggested for this disorder are prenatal (genetics/uterine environment, brain structure and function), perinatal (birth trauma) and postnatal (vaccination = MMR, food intolerance) (Gates 2007).

The word 'autism' was first used by a Boston physician called Leo Kanner in 1943. There are three main characteristics forming the triad of social communication of this disorder:

1   Social interaction – poor eye contact and use of gestures and facial expressions. These children have no interest in others or joining in. They cannot understand the effect of their behaviour on others and have no insight into their own or others' behaviour.

2   Communication – there is delay in speech. These children child misinterpret sarcasm, jokes and non-verbal cues. They also take things literally.

3   These children have restrictive, repetitive patterns of behaviour, interests and activities. They are excessive in rituals and routines and have unusual interests. These children can be prone to self-injury e.g. head banging or biting.

Autism appears in a 4:1 ratio of males to females, and Asperger's in a 10:1 ratio. They can be co-morbid with:

- learning disability;
- epilepsy;
- speech and language difficulties;
- ADHD;
- dyspraxia (motor coordination problem);
- tics and Tourette's syndrome;
- feeding and eating difficulties (refusal, hoarding, overeating) (www.nas.org.uk).

Parents are usually the first to note that their child's development is unusual and may feel relief to know there is a reason/diagnosis. However, it should not be underestimated that having a child with autistic spectrum disorder (like other disorders) can cause considerable stress in raising a child. There are three main factors that are particularly stressful: societal lack of understanding (stigma and challenging behaviour), poor service provision (pre-school and school provision), and the permanency of the condition (relationships and work). However, there is an emerging political movement of autistic people which is gaining media attention in the hope that society will alter its attitudes towards autistic spectrum disorder (Brown 2005; Gates 2007).

Prior to the inclusion of Asperger's disorder in the DSM, there was considerable controversy regarding differential diagnoses among disorders and syndromes that share common features, such as autism, Asperger's syndrome, and semantic pragmatic disorder. Even though these disorders now sit within a spectrum of pervasive developmental disorders it remains difficult to distinguish between Asperger's disorder and 'high-functioning autism' (25 per cent of children with autism), as they share similar features of social disability due to poor understanding of the pragmatics of social communication, inability to read social cues, and poor understanding of non-verbal social indicators (Wilmshurst 2004). A recent development toward a more reliable assessment tool is the Asperger Syndrome Diagnostic Scale (Smith *et al.* 2003).

Down's syndrome

Biography
British physician **John Langdon Down** (1828–1896) first described the abnormality of the twenty-first chromosome in 1866; hence the name Down's syndrome.

The most common chromosomal disorder leading to a learning disability is Down's syndrome. The overall incidence of Down's syndrome is approximately 1:600 births. Less than one of every 1000 live births results in Down's syndrome, in women aged 25 and younger. The incidence substantially increases in mothers over the age of 35 years: in mothers of 40 and over the risk rises to 1:100 and rises steeply thereafter. Definitive diagnosis is only available by blood test at 10–12 weeks, called chorionic villous sampling and at week 16 by amniocentesis.

Types of chromosomal abnormality resulting in Down's syndrome:

- Trisomy 21 accounts for 94 per cent of people with Down's syndrome. The individual has three instead of two twenty-first chromosomes.
- Translocation – the individual has two normal twenty-first chromosomes and a third twenty-first chromosome fused with another chromosome (15th or 13th).
- Mosaicism – this is extremely rare, and involves cells with two and cells with three twenty-first chromosomes found in the same person.

Down's syndrome

Signs and symptoms
- IQ between 35 and 49 (level of intellectual impairment differs in individuals)
- May have difficulty with pronunciation due to protruding tongue and intellectual disability
- May develop slower than expected milestones
- This child will age quickly so may look older than his biological age
- May develop dementia in older age (40–50) due to genes of dementia being located close to each other on chromosome 21 (ongoing research)
- Facial features = small head, flattened facial appearance, high cheek bones, hair is dry and sparse
- Congenital heart disease affects around 40 per cent
- Thyroid disease occurs in about 20 per cent (Comer 2004; Gates 2007)

Useful website: www.downs-syndrome.org.uk

Many different characteristics are associated with Down's syndrome, but it should be noted that not all children and adults with this condition will exhibit them all.

Stop and think – You are in a prime position to notice differences and atypical behaviour in terms of a child's development. Some things to think about:

- A child may not be developing according to the age and expected stage of development; this is where your knowledge of the well child and stages/ranges of development will be very useful.
- You need to pick up cues from the carer and from the response that you get from the child when communicating with her. (For ideas on communication see Chapter 3.)

> • Make sure you collect whatever enables the child to maximize his ability if possible and most certainly allow the child to take her comfort e.g. toy, doll, blanket. Remember that this child may have an 'unusual' interest in an object, such as the batteries to a toy as opposed to the toy, for example.

How to relate to a child/adult with learning disability

Children and adults with learning disability, as with the rest of the population, will display a range of behaviour. As an ambulance clinician/healthcare professional you will need to use your acute assessment and communication skills in order to establish a rapport and maximize communication with the child/adult/family/carer as soon as possible. This is in order that you get the best from them and they trust your professional care. As a healthcare professional you will use the clues around you, in terms of their living situation and how their carer communicates with them, to determine how you should communicate with them, in either a child-like or adult-like manner. Children can show challenging behaviour towards you; indeed, this can be a characteristic of a child with learning disability such as ADHD or autism. You would be wise to gain the assistance of the carer who will know how best to manage the child. In contrast, one of the most endearing (or possibly awkward, depending on your personal experience) characteristics of children with Down's syndrome, for example, is their loving nature and very often public demonstration of the same.

 Stop and think – While children with Down's syndrome are generally happy and loving and are often keen to express their love (even to strangers), this can be a disadvantage as they can be vulnerable.

You may be called to a person with learning disability who lives alone, in a supported community, with carers or with family as back-up support. Observing the environment in which the person lives may provide you with clues about how independent she may be. If a person with learning disability lives in a supported community, it is likely that she may have been encouraged with and taught some social and practical skills to enable her to live relatively independently. If, however, a person with learning disability lives with his family it may be that he is unable to live independently or has not been given the opportunity to do so.

People with learning disability who have been socialized to be more independent may have been taught to curb their affections with strangers. However, in general terms, if a person, especially a child, with learning disability takes a liking to your personable nature she will generally cooperate with you in your assessment and possibly even treatment. In contrast, if a child or adult with learning disability does not want to cooperate, she can be extremely stubborn and possibly obstructive. It is always in your best interest as a professional carer to err on the patient's good side.

Conclusion

Researchers, along with families of children with these disorders and in fact children/ adults with learning disability themselves, are speaking out about their experiences and making waves in changing how they are viewed by society. 'Nothing about us, without us' is the phrase which sums up the movement of people that have broken away from inactive involvement to directing the research that affects theirs and their children's lives. People with learning disabilities are increasingly speaking up for themselves. They want the same chances and opportunities that people without learning disabilities have. Many people with learning disabilities have successfully passed exams in school and college; they drive cars and have paid employment while living independently and forming strong relationships. This happens because they look for opportunities, they are supported if they need it and they believe change is possible (Gates 2007). There are many positive changes that have occurred in the care of children and adults with learning disabilities. However, changes need to continue to happen if this group is to be included, valued and afforded an equal status in society.

In the introduction I stated my wish that you would read this chapter and find it of interest; I hope you are pleased you didn't skip it. This chapter has provided you with a brief overview of the different approaches to child development and tried to relate these to your everyday practice of caring for children and their parents/carers. This chapter also considered atypical development to provide you with an overview of the diversity of children and young adults and their needs.

Chapter key points

- The work of many influential leaders in developmental psychology remains relevant in the twenty-first century.

- An understanding of the work of the key theorists will aid the ambulance clinician to understand more about the development and behaviour of clients requiring their care and treatment.

- In addition to 'normal' development, the ambulance clinician also requires an understanding of atypical development, in order to provide holistic care to the patient.

- Changes need to continue to happen for people with learning disability if this group is to be included, valued and afforded an equal status in society.

References, suggested reading and useful websites

Achenbach, T. (2003) *Assess Adaptive and Maladaptive Functioning. Achenbach System of Empirically Based Assessment (ASEBA)*. London: Harcourt Press.

Ainsworth, M.D.S. (1979) Infant–mother attachment, *American Psychologist*, 34: 932–7.

American Psychiatric Association (2000) *Diagnostic and Statistical Manual of Mental Disorders, DSM IV*. Philadelphia, PA: American Psychiatric Association.

Atkinson, R.L., Atkinson, R.C., Smith, E.E. and Bem, D.J. (1993) *Introduction to Psychology*, 11th edn. London: Harcourt Brace College Publishers.

Baillargeon, R., Spelkes, E.S. and Wasserman, S. (1985) Object permanence in 5-month-old infancy, *Cognition*, 20: 191–208.

Bandura, A. (1977) *Social Learning Theory*. London: Prentice-Hall.

Bandura, A. (1986) *Social Foundations of Thought and Action: A Social Cognitive Theory*. London: Prentice-Hall.

Baron-Cohen, S. and Bolton, P. (1996) *Autism: The Facts*. Buckingham: Open University Press.

Berger, K. S. (2003) *The Developing Person through Childhood and Adolescence*. New York: Worth Publishers.

Berk, L. E. (2003) *Development through the Lifespan*. London: Pearson Education.

Berryman, J., Ockleford, E., Howells, K., Hargreaves, D. and Wildbur, D. (2006) *Psychology and You. An Informal Introduction*, 3rd edn. Oxford: British Psychological Society and Blackwell Publishing.

Berryman, J.C., Smyth, P.K., Taylor, A., Lemont, A., and Joiner, R. (2002) *Developmental Psychology and You*. Oxford: British Psychological Society and Blackwell Publishing.

Bowen, M. (1994) *Piaget*. London: Fontana.

Bowlby, J. (1979) *Attachment and Loss. Volume 1: Attachment*. Harmondsworth: Penguin.

Boyle, M. (1996) *Fetal Assessment: An Overview*. Hale: Books for Midwives Press.

Bremner, G. and Slater, A. (2004) *Theories of Infant Development*. Oxford: Blackwell Publishing.

Bremner, J.G. (1994) *Infancy*. London: Blackwall Publishers.

Brown, J. (2005) Say it loud, autistic and proud, *Observer*, 30 November.

Bruce, T. and Meggitt, C. (2003) *Child Care and Education*. London: Hodder and Stoughton

Butterworth, G. and Harris, M. (1994) *Principles of Developmental Psychology*. Hove: Lawrence Erlbaum Associates.

Carpendale, J. and Lewis, C. (2006) *How Children Develop Social Understanding*. Oxford: Blackwell Publishing.

Comer, R. J. (2004) *Abnormal Psychology*, 5th edn. New York: Worth.

Davenport, G.C. (2002) *An Introduction to Child Development*. London: Collins Educational.

DoH (2000) *Framework for the Assessment of Children in Need and Their Families*. London: TSO.

Donaldson, M. (1978) *Children's Minds*. London: Fontana.

Durkin, K. (1995) *Developmental Social Psychology: From Infancy to Old Age*. Oxford: Blackwell Publishers.

Eysenck, H. J. (2000) *Psychology: A Student's Handbook*. Hove: Psychology Press.

Gates, B. (2007) *Learning Disabilities: Towards Inclusion*, 5th edn. London: Churchill Livingstone.

Gittins, D. (1998) *The Child in Question*. London: Macmillan.

Goswami, U. (1998) *Developmental Psychology: A Module Course. Cognition in Children*. London: Psychology Press Publications.

Hardy, S., Kramer, R., Holt, G., Woodward, P. and Chaplin, E. (2006) *Supporting Complex Needs: A Practical Guide for Support Staff Working with People with a Learning Disability Who Have Mental Health Needs*. London: Turning Point.

Harlow, H.F., Harlow, M.K. and Suomi, S.J. (1971) From thought to theory. Lessons from a primate laboratory, *American Scientist*, 59: 538–49.

Hewstone, M., Fincham, F.D. and Foster, J. (2005) *Psychology*. Oxford: British Psychological Society and Blackwell Publishing.

HM Government (1991) *United Nations Convention on the Rights of the Child*. London: TSO.

JRCALC (Joint Royal Colleges Ambulance Liaison Committee) (2006) *UK Ambulance Service Clinical Practice Guidelines*. London: JRCALC/Ambulance Service Association (ASA).

Keenan, T. (2002) *An Introduction to Child Development*. London: Sage Publications.

Klin, A., Sparrow, S.S., Volkmar, F.R., Ciccetti, D.V. and Rourke, B.T. (1995) Asperger's syndrome, in B.P. Rourke (ed.) *Syndrome of Nonverbal Learning Disabilities: Neurodevelopment Manifestations.* New York: Guildford.

Kroger, J. (2000) *Identity Development: Adolescent through Adulthood.* London: Sage Publications.

Lechte, J. (2004) *Fifty Key Contemporary Thinkers. From Structuralism to Postmodernity.* Oxford: Routledge.

Lee, V. and Das Gupta, P. (1995) *Children's Cognitive and Language Development.* London: Blackwell/Open University Press.

Maynard, T. and Thomas, N. (2005) *An Introduction to Early Childhood Studies.* London: Sage Publications.

Messer, D. and Mill, S. (1999) *Exploring Developmental Psychology from Infant to Adolescent.* London: Arnold Publishers.

Montgomery, H., Burr, R. and Woodhead, M. (2003) *Changing Childhoods: Local and Global.* Chichester: Wiley.

Morton, J. (2004) *Understanding Developmental Disorders: A Causal Modelling Approach.* Oxford: Blackwell Publishing.

Muuss R.E. (1996) *Theories of Adolescence,* 6th edn. London: McGraw-Hill.

Palmer, J.A. (2004) *Fifty Major Thinkers on Education. From Confucius to Dewey.* Oxford: Routledge.

Palmer, J.A. (2005) *Fifty Modern Thinkers on Education. From Piaget to Present.* Oxford: Routledge.

Pavlov, I.P. (1927) *Conditioned Reflexes.* Oxford: Oxford University Press.

Payne, S. and Walker, J. (2000) *Psychology for Nurses and the Caring Professions.* Buckingham: OU Press.

Piaget, J. and Inhelder, B. (1967) *The Psychology of the Child.* London: Routledge.

Pugh, G. and Duffy, B. (2007) *Contemporary Issues in the Early Years,* 4th edn. London: Sage Publications.

Richardson, K. (2000) *Developmental Psychology: How Nature and Nurture Interact.* London: Macmillan.

Royal College of Psychiatrists (2001) *Diagnostic Criteria for Psychiatric Disorders for Use with Adults with Learning Disabilities/Mental Retardation.* Occasional paper OP48. London: Gaskell.

Schaffer, H.R. (2006) *Key Concepts in Development Psychology.* London: Sage Publications.

Sheridan, M.D., Cockerill, H. and Sharma, A. (2007) *From Birth to Five Years. Children's Developmental Progress.* Oxford: Elsevier.

Smith, P.K., Cowie, H. and Blades, M. (2003) *Understanding Children's Development,* 4th edition. Oxford: Blackwell.

Vygotsky, L. (1962) *Thought and Language.* Boston, MA: MIT Press.

Wenar, C. and Kerig, P. (2000) *Developmental Psychopathology: From Infancy through Adolescence.* Boston, MA: McGraw-Hill.

Wilmshurst, L. (2004) *Child and Adolescent Psychopathology: A Casebook.* London: Sage Publications.

Wood, C., Littleton, K. and Sheehy, K. (2006) *Developmental Psychology in Action.* Milton Keynes: Open University Press.

Wood, D. (1998) *How Children Think and Learn,* 2nd edn. Oxford: Blackwell.

Zimbardo, P., McDermott M., Jansz, J. and Metaal, N. (1995) *Psychology: A European Text.* London: Harper Collins Publishers Ltd.

Useful websites

The Down's Syndrome Organisation is the only organisation within the UK focusing solely on all aspects of living with Down's Syndrome. It has been established since 1970 and has grown from being a local parent support group to a national charity with over 20,000 members: www.downs-syndrome.org.uk

Estia Centre is a training, research and development resource for those who support adults with learning disabilities and additional mental health needs: estiacentre.org

For free downloads of the books listed below in pdf format, see www.estiacentre.org/freepub.html

Mental Health, a charity aiming to improve the lives of those with mental health problems or learning disability: www.mentalhealth.org.uk

MIND is a leading charity in England and Wales working to create a better life for anyone with experience of mental distress: www.mind.org.uk

The National Autistic Society champions the rights and interests of all people with autism and aims to provide individuals with autism and their families with help, support and services: www.nas.org.uk

Turning Point is the UK's leading social care organization providing services for people with complex needs, including those affected by drug and alcohol misuse, mental health problems and those with a learning disability: www.turning-point.co.uk

8

Abnormal psychology: an introduction
Jackie Whitnell

Topics covered:

- Introduction
- Why is this relevant?
- Child and Adolescent Mental Health (CAMH)
- Depression
- Eating problems
- Anxiety
- An overview of behavioural disturbance
- Mental Health Act 1983/2007/Mental Capacity Act 2005
- Conclusion
- Chapter key points
- References, suggested reading and useful websites

Introduction

> ### Definition of abnormal psychology
> The scientific studies of abnormal behaviour in order to describe, predict, explain, and change abnormal patterns of functioning (Comer 2004: 3).

Abnormal psychology focuses on the causes and treatment of psychological disorders and adjustment problems, such as depression and phobias (colloquially referred to as 'mental health problems' or 'mental ill health'). Estimates of the prevalence of mental distress in Britain vary. The Office for National Statistics (ONS) (2000, 2006a, 2006b) (previously the Office for Population Censuses and Surveys or OPCS) puts the figure at one in six adults at any one time. The one in six figures given by the ONS

(2006a) represents those people defined as having 'significant' mental health problems. Mental health problems are common at all ages, affecting one in four people at
some point in their life. Mental health problems vary from anxiety, phobia and mild
depression to more serious disorders such as severe depression and schizophrenia,
which can be recurrent, remitting and enduring. Disturbed behaviour falls into three
categories:

1   *Situational = Exogenous.* This person is in crisis. He either has coping strategies to
    reduce the crisis or escape, such as using alcohol, drugs or induced psychiatric
    symptoms, or will deliberately self-harm and/or commit suicide.
2   *Organic = Somatic.* This disturbed behaviour is possibly due to physical illness/
    disease state such as diabetes, alcohol, drugs, delirium, dementia.
3   *Psychiatric = Endogenous.* This person may be suffering from psychotic disorders
    such as schizophrenia or anxiety disorders, or affective disorders e.g. depression
    (Comer 2004).

The frequency of mental health problems is well documented statistically. However,
these figures need to be treated with some caution. Often widely differing figures will
be given for the same mental health problem, making it difficult to determine exactly
how common it is. This is partly because these figures are not always measuring the
same thing. For example, in order to reflect the fact that mental health is not fixed but
likely to change over time, a variety of different figures are used. The most common
are:

Prevalence: this measures the number of people with a particular diagnosis at a given
time.

Lifetime prevalence: this measures the number of people who have experienced a
particular mental health problem at any time in their lives.

Incidence: this measures the number of new cases of a particular mental health
problem that appear in a given time period.

Often these figures are compared to provide further information about a mental
health problem. For example, comparing the number of new cases (the incidence)
with the number who are ill at any one time (the prevalence) can give us a rough idea
of the average amount of time a mental health problem is likely to last.

Another important factor is the kind of sample used to arrive at a particular
figure. Often the number of people treated by health professionals is used to determine how common a mental health problem is. However, this is likely to ignore all
those who have not come into contact with services. Furthermore, psychiatric diagnosis is often far from straightforward – a person's diagnosis may be changed several
times in the course of her treatment.

Mental health problems may be associated with, provoked and maintained by
alcohol or other substances, possibly making the care of these individuals difficult.
Indeed, while some patients will volunteer to accept your help, others will not and may

need to be compelled to receive an assessment and treatment, possibly against their will using the powers of legislation (DoH 1983, 2007; JRCALC 2006).

Due to the introductory nature of this text, this chapter will provide the reader with a brief overview of mental ill health. The chapter will commence with an overview on Child and Adolescent Mental Health; statistically this is an issue that has been raised in the public profile in recent years (DfES 2003). The chapter will continue with discussion on some relatively common mental health problems/disorders that the ambulance clinician is likely to encounter in contact with patients during their working practice.

Why is this relevant?

It is extremely important that healthcare professionals have at least an understanding of some of the most common mental illnesses from which people may suffer, and an idea of some of the signs and symptoms that the client/patient may exhibit. Ambulance clinicians will be in the position of caring for people with mental health problems and will make assessments during their working practice. It is the intention that this overview will at least provide some information and excite an interest and thirst for further exploration of this area of ill health.

Child and Adolescent Mental Health (CAMH)

There are a wide range of mental health problems that can affect children and adolescents. In 2004, the results from the Office for National Statistics on the mental health needs of children and young people were published (Green et al. 2004). One in 10 children (10 per cent) aged 5 to 16 years have a mental disorder which is clinically recognizable based on the International Classification of Disease Related Health Problems (ICD-10) which is a classification of mental and behavioural disorders with strict impairment criteria. Latest statistics from the 2004 survey found that 4 per cent of children suffered with emotional disorders such as anxiety or depression, 6 per cent with conduct disorders (Hasnie 2007), 2 per cent with hyperkinetic disorders such as Attention Deficit Hyperactive Disorder and 1 per cent from less common disorders including autism and eating disorders. Two per cent of children suffer from more than one type of disorder; this poses a greater challenge in terms of diagnosis and also in the care of the child (Green et al. 2004). The incidence of behavioural problems and conduct disorders is estimated to be 10–20 per cent. In a hypothetical secondary school of 1000 pupils there are likely to be 50 young people who are seriously depressed and at risk of deliberately self-harming, which occurs in 3 per cent of the teenage population. Hyperactivity, in its extreme form, affects between 10 and 20 per cent of children. Attention Deficit Hyperactivity Disorder is estimated to affect 2–5 per cent of children. Severe eating disorder affects about 1 per cent of teenage girls (DfES 2004).

Link to Chapter 7 Read the section on atypical development for more information on the conditions mentioned above.

 Stop and think – Before continuing, jot down some of the risk factors for mental health problems in children and young people.

The Audit Commission (1999) identified a number of environmental, family and individual factors that can lead to a higher level of risk of mental health problems in children and young people. These include living in families where the main 'bread-winner' is unemployed, having a parent with a mental illness, and having some form of learning disability. Other possible causes are genetic predisposition, stress at home or school, over-protective parents and an over-controlling environment.

The Audit Commission (1999) estimated that 80 per cent of children and adolescents with mental health problems are also likely to experience family life and relationship difficulties. Thankfully, suicide is rare in childhood and early adolescence, but it becomes more frequent with increasing age. The latest mean world-wide annual rates of suicide per 100,000 were 0.5 for females and 0.9 for males among 5- to 14-year-olds and 12.0 for females and 14.2 for males among 15- to 24-year-olds. The relationship between psychiatric disorders and adolescent suicide is now well established. Prior suicide attempts, mood disorders and substance misuse are strongly related (Pelkonen and Marttunen 2003).

Depression

The criteria for depressive disorders are the same or similar for children and adults (depression in adults will be discussed further on in this chapter). However, there are differences in how this disorder shows itself for different ages. In children, the type of depression is called dysthmia, characterized by a chronically depressed mood for at least a year, with irritability (Achenbach 2003).

Dysthmia (depression)

Signs and symptoms for differing ages:

Infant/toddler – loss of developmentally appropriate behaviour e.g. toilet training and intellectual function.

Pre-school – sad appearance, regress to earlier development e.g. separation anxiety and sleep problems.

School age – able to express their feelings; more like adults. Eating and sleep disturbances, self-critical, low motivation.

In terms of gender and depression in childhood, it is similar for girls and boys. In puberty, however, there are more girls than boys that suffer with depression and the same into adulthood. Girls internalize their feelings, whereas boys externalize their feelings. Consequently, one could argue that as girls express this disorder more in their mood outwardly it is more noticeable and easier to detect. One approach used to explain the occurrence of depression in childhood derives from the attachment theory (Bowlby 1969). This theory suggests that insecure attachment can lead to depression in infants, children and adolescents. Feeling insecure leads to unworthiness and the feeling of being unloved can predispose children to being vulnerable, fearing disapproval and abandonment. A further consideration from the social-cultural theory suggests the cause could derive from problems in the home, in school or with peers (Berger 2003; Smith *et al.* 2003).

Depression

Signs and symptoms

- Sadness
- Tired
- Self-pity
- Loss of appetite
- Disturbed sleep pattern
- Thoughts of death

Eating problems

According to the Mental Health Foundation (1997), current estimates suggest that up to 1 per cent of women in the UK between the ages of 15 and 30 suffer from anorexia nervosa, and between 1 and 2 per cent suffer from bulimia nervosa. These figures are likely to be much higher, as many cases of eating disorder are unreported or undiagnosed. Eating disorders are much more likely to occur among women than men. However, for anorexia, there is also evidence to suggest that in the younger age group (7–14 years), up to 25 per cent of cases are boys.

Anxiety

Anxiety appears to involve cognition, physiological problems, emotion and behaviour. The child/young person can perceive extreme danger or fear (cognition), then experience symptoms like nausea, sweating and dizziness (physiological) and then feel scared and anxious (emotion), and tries to avoid the situation or is unable to function (behaviour).

Link to Chapter 6 for further discussion on the case study of Shaun.

There are different types of anxiety, for example:

- specific phobias;
- obsessive–compulsive disorder (boys > girls);
- separation anxiety disorder;
- social phobia;
- panic disorder (girls > boys).

These will be discussed in more detail further in this chapter.

Stop and think – You may experience a child or person who suffers from anxiety; how would you approach this person? How would you try to calm the child/adult in order to care for them and transport them safely?

When children and young people present with mental health problems, the solution to their difficulties is rarely straightforward. The Audit Commission (1999) states that only 5 per cent of children present with one problem, the most frequent number of problems being five, while half of children referred to Child and Adolescent Mental Health (CAMH) services have at least two severe problems (co-morbid). The *Every Child Matters* agenda (DfES 2003) is trying to ensure the well-being of children and young people through mental health promotion and the Children's Commissioner for England has launched a new website calling for children and young people to get involved. The new website is called www.11million.org.uk and is a new interactive website. A group of children and young people with direct experience of mental health issues are working with '11 Million', sharing their experiences and opinions and helping to shape the organization's work.

As an ambulance clinician you will transport children and adolescents with mental health problems. It is important that you have a good understanding of the types of issues and difficulties facing these children as well as report your findings of the interactions you observe between the child/young person and significant others, noting anything that you find unusual, inappropriate or unsafe.

An overview of behavioural disturbance

Suicide and self-harm

Definitions of suicide

Suicide is the taking of one's own life (www.healthline.com).
A self-inflicted death in which one makes an intentional, direct and conscious effort to end one's own life (Shneidman 1985).

Without doubt, there is no greater problem facing mental health practitioners than suicide-related behaviour. Since the mid 1970s the data gathered has consistently indicated that suicide is a leading cause of death in young people. The possible contributing factors could include decriminalization of the suicide act in 1961, drug prescribing increase since the 1960s, better emergency procedures and resuscitation methods and the rise in unemployment at the end of the 1970s and early 1990s. In 2005, there were 5671 suicides in adults aged 15 years and over in the UK, which represented 1 per cent of all adult deaths. Almost three-quarters of these suicides were among men, and this division between the sexes was broadly similar throughout the period 1991–2005 (Office for National Statistics 2003; www.statistics.gov.uk).

Suicide rates for men are higher than for women in all age groups, and currently men are almost three times more likely than women to commit suicide. This gender gap has widened considerably over the past few decades: in 1979 the female to male gender ratio for suicides was 2:3 and in 2002 it was around 1:3. This difference is particularly striking for young people, with males between 25 and 34 almost four times more likely than women to kill themselves. The group at highest risk of suicide used to be males aged over 65 years of age: 24 per 100,000 population in 1979. In the past decade, the group at highest risk was males aged 25–34 years. Suicide is the most common cause of death among men aged between 15 and 44 years (www.statistics.gov.uk). Young females in the 15–24 age group are at the lowest risk. The suicide rate for this group has remained fairly constant since 1979, and is now around three per 100,000 population. Currently, the data indicates that in some areas suicide is increasing in men between 35 and 44 years and women 25–34 years. The highest increase has been for older women, aged 75+. For this group, the figure has gone up from six suicides per 100,000 population in 2001 to eight suicides per 100,000 population in 2002 (Samaritans 2004).

The likelihood of a person committing suicide depends on many factors: social problems – especially those related to family stress, separation, divorce, social isolation, death of a loved one and unemployment (an unemployed man is two to three times more at risk of suicide than the general population); mental and physical illness; access to the means of suicide. Other factors that can increase the risk of suicide are cultural issues (women born in India and East Africa have a 40 per cent higher suicide rate than those born in England and Wales; Roy 1996), homelessness and mental health problems (Craig and Hodson 1996; Samaritans 2004). Certain occupational groups such as doctors, nurses, pharmacists, vets and farmers are at higher risk of suicide. This is partly because of ease of access to the means of suicide. Marital status affects a person's risk of suicide. Among men under 45 years old, the increase in suicides between the early 1970s and late 1980s has been linked to more men remaining single or becoming divorced. Alcohol and drug use are also factors which can influence suicide risk. Men are known to have far higher drug and alcohol consumption rates than women, and the figures are particularly high for younger men.

Suicide by self-poisoning is an important cause of death worldwide. A substantial proportion of those with a fatal outcome may come into contact with an ambulance clinician and/or emergency department before they die. A multicentre study by Kapur *et al.* (2005) found that the UK might expect 300 self-poisoning suicides per year to reach hospital alive (6 per cent of all suicides).

The incidence of self-harm, which has always been high, does not seem to be abating. Some professionals argue that attempted suicide and self-harm are both the same entity; it is put forward that they are two sides of the same coin and this coin is termed 'suicide-related behaviour' (Bird and Faulkner 2000).

The term 'suicide-related behaviour' is a general term used to describe all behaviours where the person intended to kill or harm himself. Deliberate self-harm is frequently encountered by ambulance clinicians and healthcare professions; it is a hidden health problem worldwide (McAllister *et al.* 2002). Approximately 4 per cent of the population will self-harm and it is one of the leading five causes of acute medical admission for women and men. Deliberate self-harm is the intentional damage to one's own body, without a conscious intent to die. The myth around self-harm is that it is a cry for attention; this is not totally accurate. While deliberate self-harm can communicate to others the pain that is inside, or that the individual needs help and is in crisis, self-harm is also commonly completed in private. It is true to say that family, friends and therapists may be unaware of the episodes of self-harm a person is experiencing (Pembroke *et al.* 1998).

Box 8.1 shows some facts and risk factors for suicide.

Box 8.1 Suicide: a serious mental health and public health problem

Facts about suicide

- Suicide occurs across the world, but rates vary by culture.
- Suicide is the most common cause of death among men aged between 15 and 44 years (www.statistics.gov.uk).
- In all cultures, men are more likely than women to complete suicide.
- Rates of suicide in children and adolescents are on the increase.
- People with mental disorders, especially depression, schizophrenia and borderline personality disorder, are at high risk for suicide.

Risk factors

- Past history of attempted suicide
- Talking about committing suicide
- A clear plan to commit suicide
- Available means (e.g. access to a gun, drugs)
- Depression
- Substance abuse
- Hopelessness
- Impulsivity
- Stressful life events
- Lack of social support
- Saying goodbye to people
- Giving away personal items

(Hewstone *et al.* 2005: 320)

An assessment tool used by ambulance clinicians in their practice is shown in Box 8.2.

Box 8.2 Suicide and self-harm risk assessment form		
Item	*Value*	*Patient score*
Sex: female	0	
Sex: male	1	
Age: less than 19 years old	1	
Age: greater than 45 years old	1	
Depression/hopelessness	1	
Previous attempts at self-harm	1	
Evidence of excess alcohol/illicit drug use	1	
Rational thinking absent	1	
Separated/divorced/widowed	1	
Organized or serious attempt	1	
No close/reliable family, job or active religious affiliation	1	
Determined to repeat or ambivalent	1	
Total patient score		
		(JRCALC 2006)

< 3 = Low risk
3–6 = Medium risk
> 6 = High risk

Anxiety disorders in adults

Definition of anxiety
An illness that produces an intense, often unrealistic and excessive state of apprehension and fear. This may or may not occur during, or in anticipation of, a specific situation, and may be accompanied by a rise in blood pressure, increased heart rate, rapid breathing, nausea and other sign of agitation or discomfort.

The Office for National Statistics (2006a) estimates that 4.7 per cent of adults experience generalized anxiety disorders (not including depression) at any one time. A further 9.2 per cent of the population have mixed anxiety and depression. Anxiety is far more common in women than in men. The prevalence of mixed anxiety and depression is 11.2 per cent in women compared to 7.2 per cent in men. Mood, stress-related and anxiety disorders are the most common groups of problems and often represent the extremes of normal emotion. They are recognized by a set of symptoms:

- Depressed mood (to be discussed further on in this chapter)
- Emotional – fear, worry

- Physical – shortness of breath, sweating, upset stomach, heart pounding
- Cognitive – fear of dying, losing control, 'going crazy'.

(American Psychiatric Association 2000)

The experience of this set of symptoms is often referred to as a 'panic attack'. Anxiety is a usual part of our everyday lives, so how do we differentiate between 'normal' or manageable fear from anxiety and impairment due to unmanageable anxiety? A disorder can be classified when there is fear and anxiety in response to something that is not inherently frightening or dangerous.

Box 8.3 Anxiety disorder

Anxiety disorders have four things in common:

- Each is defined by a specific target of fear (the situation/item the person is afraid of).
- Anxiety or panic attacks are experienced in response to the target of fear.
- The target of fear is avoided by the sufferer.
- Anxiety disorders tend to be chronic – they tend to persist rather than being episodic.

(Hewstone *et al.* 2005: 326)

Types of anxiety disorder

1   *Specific phobias* – fear and avoidance of a particular object or situation (e.g. dogs, heights, flying). People can live a *normal* life, by avoiding their phobia, unless they are asked to confront their fear.

2   *Social phobia* – tends to be more impairing as it involves significant social isolation. People with this type of phobia are afraid of rejection and negative evaluation, so they avoid it at all costs. These phobias can be mild (fearing public speaking – link to case study of Shaun in Chapter 7) or severe (fearing all social interaction). The Office for National Statistics (2006a) found that 1.9 per cent of adults in Britain experience phobias and women are twice as likely as men to suffer.

3   *Panic disorder* – can be debilitating, especially when accompanied by agoraphobia.

Definition of agoraphobia

Fear of situations in which escape would be difficult or help is not available should panic or anxiety occur (Hewstone *et al.* (2005: 327).

Panic disorders are related to anxiety. According to the ONS study (2006a), seven people per 1000 develop a panic disorder and this appears to be the same across all age groups and roughly the same for men and women, with a female to male ratio of

7:8. The anxiety begins with panic attacks that occur *out of the blue*. The disorder gets worse when people worry about having another panic attack and begin to avoid places and situations associated with the panic attack. However, panic disorder is the least common form of mental distress according to the ONS survey.

- *Obsessive-compulsive disorder* (OCD) – can be quite specific, but can also cause domination and impairment of someone's life. Typical compulsions are hand washing, checking, counting and hoarding. It is traditionally regarded as a neurotic disorder, like phobias and anxiety states (De Silva and Rachmann 1998).

  Around 1.2 per cent of the population of Britain have OCD at any one time (ONS 2000) This statistic is up by 0.5 per cent from the 1993 survey. The ONS (2006a) survey gives a female to male ratio of 15:9.

Definitions

Obsessions – Unwanted, persistent, intrusive, repetitive thoughts (Hewstone *et al.* 2005: 327).

Compulsions – Ritualistic, repetitive behaviours that a person feels compelled to engage in (Hewstone *et al.* 2005: 327).

- *Post-traumatic stress disorder* – see specific section below.
- *Generalized anxiety disorder* – is characterized by a period of over six months of chronic, uncontrollable worry about numerous things. Sufferers are worried and tense at all times, easily irritated and have trouble sleeping and concentrating.

Post-traumatic stress disorder (PTSD)

Is one of the anxiety disorders, but is worthy of specific attention due to the nature of the role of an ambulance clinician.

 Stop and think – Consider the local and global situations that people have found themselves in over recent years that may predispose to a person suffering from PTSD.

PTSD was first noted among war veterans. It can be equally seen in victims of trauma and in observers who witness or are involved in the event. Stress is the cause of PTSD. Up to 30 per cent of people experience a traumatic event in their life which may develop into PTSD.

It can present in children following a traumatic event such as experiencing the divorce of their parents, seeking asylum, child abuse and/or living with domestic abuse. Globally people are migrating and seeking asylum: refugees are a vulnerable group. PTSD sufferers have a high suicide rate.

Post-traumatic stress disorder

Signs and symptoms/presentation
Paradoxical symptoms:

- Fear of the trauma itself creates anxiety so the person will avoid anything associated with the trauma (avoidance).
- May lose their memory for the event, or be plagued with intrusive and unwanted thoughts, such as flashbacks and nightmares (re-experience).
- People tend to be psychologically numb, emotionally 'shut down', find no pleasure in things and cannot look to the future (emotional numbing).
- Conversely the person may have symptoms of 'hyper-arousal' – startle easily, cannot sleep or concentrate, irritable and easily angered.

Specific recognition for children and young people.

- Do not rely wholly on an adult's assessment; ask the child or young person to explain.
- Ask the adult/child about sleep patterns or significant changes to it.

(www.niceguidance)

Depression

Definition of depression

Common cold of psychopathology (Seligman 1973b).

Depression with anxiety is experienced by 9.2 per cent of people in Britain, and depression without anxiety by 2.8 per cent. Overall, depression occurs in 1 in 10 adults or 10 per cent of the population in Britain at any one time (ONS 2000). One in six adults living in Great Britain have a neurotic disorder (anxiety, depression). One in seven adults have considered suicide at some point in their lives. One in 200 has a psychotic disorder i.e. psychosis and/or schizophrenia. All neurotic disorders are more common in women than men, except panic disorder, which is equal for both. Women have a higher prevalence of mixed anxiety and depressive disorder than men: the ONS figure for women is 11.2 per cent of the population and for men 7.2 per cent. However, recent studies suggest depression occurs as often in men, though women are twice as likely to be diagnosed and treated. It is argued that men tend to express their symptoms differently, for example through the use of alcohol and drugs, and are unwilling to admit to the symptoms of depression. It is therefore interesting to note that the figures for men are rising faster than the figures for women. This may indicate that men now are more likely to admit to feeling depressed (Stewart 2005).

Mood disorders may have some common symptoms but they have very different causes and prevalence to other disorders. Unipolar depression or major depressive disorder is one of the most common. Less prevalent are the bipolar disorders (otherwise known as manic depression) and psychotic disorders such as schizophrenia. Depression is a disorder that affects people of all age groups, including children. The age onset of major depressive disorder is reducing; early onset predicts a worse course of depression over time. Depression follows a recurrent course. Most people have multiple episodes that become worse with time, while some may have isolated episodes. Mild depression with a few symptoms may indicate the person will suffer with more serious depression later on. The feelings of major depressive disorder should not be negated. Fifteen per cent of depressed people commit suicide, due to the feelings of hopelessness and long-term suffering (Clark and Goebel-Fabbri in Hewstone *et al.* 2005).

Unipolar depression

Signs and symptoms/presentation
Primary symptom is sad or depressed mood, but it is much more than this. Other symptoms include:

- Lack of interest or pleasure in things that are usually enjoyed
- Changes in appetite
- Changes in sleep habits
- Low level of energy, poor concentration and extreme fatigue
- Feeling bad about themselves, low self-esteem, negative self-concept; self-reproach and blaming themselves for what has 'gone wrong' in their life, 'paralysis of will' (Beck 1967)
- Hopelessness about the future
- Preoccupation with ailments and death – suicidal ideation

Bipolar disorder: commonly known as manic depression

Most studies give a lifetime prevalence of 1 per cent for bipolar disorder and equal prevalence rates for men and women. Bipolar is a common health problem affecting between 1 and 2 per cent of the population and it affects people of all ages. However, hospital admission rates are much higher owing to the recurrent nature of the illness. It is a serious mental illness, but if it is well managed with help from family, friends, support groups and health professionals, then a person with bipolar can lead a productive and satisfying life (www.bbc.co.uk/health; www.nice.org.uk). However, if left untreated one in seven people with the diagnosis will commit suicide. Manic depression has no known cure; a person may require psychiatric treatment for the rest of her life, although it is estimated that 20 per cent of people who have a first episode of manic depression do not get another (www.mind.org.uk). It is considered that sufferers of bipolar depression have a predisposition genetically, but the manic state can be triggered by the stresses and strains of everyday life, or a traumatic event. Sufferers experience sudden onset lasting anything from one or two days to weeks or months. The average age of people with bipolar used to be 32 years, but in the last decade it has dropped to under 19 years of age.

Bipolar disorder

Signs and symptoms/presentation

- Highs and lows are increasingly disconnected from everyday events and out of control
- People feel excessively self-important, expansive and over-confident with inflated self-esteem or grandiose ideas
- Increase in goal-directed activity
- May become sexually promiscuous, excessively religious, financially irresponsible, intolerant, verbally aggressive, irritable, over-communicative and incapable of listening to or empathizing with other people
- May suffer from hallucinations, delusions and paranoia in extreme depression
- May suffer from sleeplessness and overactive behaviour (www.bbc.co.uk/health)
- Occurs in 1% of the population. Unipolar disorder occurs in 17% of the population, so is more prevalent than bipolar disorder.

The symptoms of this disorder may only be spotted with the onset of a severe crisis in a person's life and may require compulsory treatment under the Mental Health Act (1983/2007). It may only be then that the person is referred to a psychiatric unit and diagnosed for treatment.

Another form of depression seen less frequently is that of postnatal depression. The most common form of postnatal disturbance is the 'baby blues', which is said to be experienced by at least half of all Western mothers. This usually lasts between 12 and 24 hours, generally occurring between the third and sixth day after the birth. This is perfectly normal and the mother and family may just need reassurance. An incidence figure of 10 per cent of all new mothers is most often quoted, with other studies showing a figure between 3 per cent and 22 per cent. It is likely that around 50 per cent of these cases will never come to medical attention. However, puerperal psychosis is a severe and relatively rare form of postnatal depression affecting between 0.1 and 0.2 per cent of all new mothers and as an ambulance clinician you may be called to a patient suffering from this, where the husband/partner/carer is very concerned about the mother's behaviour (Comer 2004).

Personality disorder

Another disorder that you may identify in a patient/client is personality disorder. This is 'an enduring pattern of inner experience and behaviour that deviates markedly from the expectations of the individual's culture, is pervasive and inflexible, has an onset in adolescence or early adulthood, is stable over time, and leads to distress or impairment' (American Psychiatric Association 2000). In Britain, the prevalence of personality disorder ranges from 2 per cent to 13 per cent according to different studies. The concept of a personality disorder is controversial and use of this diagnosis is often questioned. Some diagnoses are applied more commonly to men (such as dissocial personality disorder), while others are applied more commonly to women (such as borderline personality disorder) (www.mind.org.uk).

Definition of personality disorder

Disorders of people's basic character structure – so there is no normal functioning to return to (Hewstone *et al.* 2005: 332).

Personality disorder

Signs and symptoms/presentation

All personality disorders have some things in common:

- Long-standing – begin at a relatively early age
- Chronic – continue over time
- Pervasive – occur in most contexts

The behaviour, thoughts and feelings seen in personality disorder are:

- Inflexible – resistant to change and are applied in a rigid manner
- Maladaptive – they do not enable the person to get what they expect/want.

Sufferers of personality disorder will generally consider the other person has the 'problem'; people with personality disorders do not think it is their 'problem'. Consequently this may lead to treatment issues. It is always wise to consider your own safety and that of your patient in difficult situations (Comer 2004).

The DSM-IV (American Psychiatric Association 2000) describes the main disorders and their traits.

There are 10 personality disorders that form three clusters:

Cluster A – the odd and eccentric cluster

- Paranoid – suspicious, distrustful, makes hostile attributions
- Schizoid – interpersonally and emotionally cut off, unresponsive to others, a 'loner'
- Schizotypal – odd thoughts, behaviours, experiences, poor interpersonal functioning

Cluster B – the dramatic and erratic cluster

- Histrionic – dramatic, wants attention, emotionally shallow
- Narcissistic – inflated sense of self-importance, will feel entitled, low empathy, hidden vulnerability
- Antisocial – behaviours that disregard laws, norms, rights of others; lacking in empathy
- Borderline – instability in thoughts, feelings, behaviour and sense of self

Cluster C – the fearful and avoidant cluster

- Obsessive-compulsive – rigid, controlled, perfectionist
- Avoidant – fears negative evaluation, rejection and abandonment
- Dependent – submissive, dependent on others for self-esteem

Personality disorders are long-term patterns of emotional functioning. Each of the 10 disorders has a low prevalence in the general population. Most people with personality disorders do not seek, want or comply with treatment, consequently treatment is not effective (Comer 2004).

 Stop and think – Consider the three clusters and think about how you would manage a person expressing these symptoms towards you, who required immediate treatment.

Psychoses

Psychoses and functional psychoses are disorders that produce disturbances in thinking and perception that are severe enough to distort the person's perception of the world and the relationship of events in it. Psychoses are normally divided into two groups:

1 Organic psychoses, such as dementia and Alzheimer's disease. Twenty per cent of people in the UK over the age of 80 years and 6 per cent over the age of 65 years are affected by dementia. There are some 683,597 people with dementia known to health authorities in the UK. Over two-thirds of them are diagnosed with Alzheimer's disease. The Alzheimer's Society reports that dementia currently affects over 700,000 individuals in the UK. By 2021, the number is expected to rise to around 940,110 (Alzheimer's Society 2007; www.alzheimers.org.uk).

2 Functional psychoses, which mainly cover schizophrenia and manic depression (although 'functional psychosis' does not necessarily have to belong to any one of these two diagnoses and can exist as a diagnosis in itself).

Schizophrenia

Definition of schizophrenia

Group of psychotic disorders characterized by the breakdown of integrated personality functioning, withdrawal from reality, emotional distortions and disturbed thought processes (Zimbardo *et al.* 1995: 642).

Schizophrenia is a complex and puzzling illness; experts in the field are not exactly sure what causes it. This is a common and often severe mental illness. It may present acutely with severe change in behaviour or insidiously as a slow but progressive change over a period of time. Some physicians think that the brain may not be able to process information correctly. Genetic factors appear to play a role, as people who have family members with schizophrenia may be more likely to inherit the disease themselves. Most studies show a lifetime prevalence for schizophrenia of just under 1 per cent, and prevalence rates of two to four per 1000 of the population (0.2–0.4 per cent) at any one time. While prevalence rates are the same for men and women, age and gender together is an important factor: one study shows incidence for men aged 15–24 years is twice that for women, whereas for those aged 24–35 years it is higher among women. This reflects a common late onset of the illness for women (Tsuang and Faraone 1998; Comer 2004).

Schizophrenia

Signs and symptoms/presentation
Any of these:

- Perceiving things that are not there – auditory hallucinations, may also be visual and tactile
- Paranoid delusions – believing things that are not true, delusions of grandeur, delusions of persecution
- Using bizarre language 'word salad' (jumbled words)
- Their behaviour may be reported by others and seriously disordered or irrational
- Lack of demonstrating emotions facially, inappropriate laughing, crying and anger

---

Behaviour disturbances can be grouped in four areas:

- Repetitive movements and mannerisms
- Significant lack of motivation – this can be termed 'avolition'
- Struggle to take care of themselves with 'basic' things such as washing or dressing
- Social withdrawal, poor social skills and strained relationships with others

All of the above symptoms can be termed either 'positive' or 'negative'. Positive symptoms describe unusual occurrences, such as hallucinations, delusions, odd speech. Negative symptoms describe the lack of behaviour that is normal for the rest of society, for example good social skills, motivation, expression of emotion and being able to look after oneself.

Schizophrenia appears to occur in equal rates among men and women, but women have a later onset. For this reason, males tend to account for more than half of patients in services with high proportions of young adults (Comer 2004). Ambulance clinicians and healthcare professionals should be aware that some of the features of schizophrenia can occur alongside the presence of physical disease, intoxication with licitly or illicitly obtained substances and/or under the influence of psychotropic drugs. It is important that you attempt to ascertain what the person may have taken in the form of drugs/substances in order that you can report it and at the same time identify risk factors to the patient/client and to yourself.

This chapter has provided the reader with a brief overview of mental ill health with consideration for the relatively common mental health problems/disorders that ambulance clinicians are likely to encounter during their working practice. This chapter will continue with information regarding the legislative powers which may be required to be used when managing the patient/client with mental ill health.

Mental Health Act 1983/2007/Mental Capacity Act 2005

The Act of 2007 was passed through parliament in July 2007; it serves to update the previous Mental Health Act of 1983. There are seven major amendments to the 1983 Act and a further eighth amendment, updating the Mental Capacity Act of 2005. The amendments provide better safeguards for mental health service users, the new rights to advocacy, a say in who their nearest relative is and the right to refuse electro-convulsive therapy and other treatments.

The Royal College of Psychiatrists is working to achieve improvements to the Code of Practice. The Department of Health have produced a draft illustrative code and a draft memorandum. The draft illustrative code is currently being updated to reflect the new Mental Health Act (2007) (www.rcpsych.ac.uk/pressparliament/mentalhealthact2007.aspx).

Criteria for application for admission under the Mental Health Act 2007

- A person suffering from a mental illness, who is either a danger to themselves or to the public, may be removed from a public place or their home to a place of safety (usually a police station or hospital) by a police officer.

As an ambulance clinician you would usually be empowered by the appropriate Approved Social Worker/Approved Mental Health Practitioner or family member to convey the patient compulsorily under Section Order to hospital. You may have to call on the services of a police officer to aid with escort or in the presence of threat of violence. It is vitally important that a bed has been secured for the patient; however, in reality it may be some time before a bed is available and the hospital may enlist the help of a psychiatric nurse while the patient remains in the Emergency Department, when the patient has been seen by the psychiatrist and is awaiting admission. Until the patient is seen by the psychiatrist, the patient remains under the Section and the police officer/s are legally obliged to stay in the Emergency Department until they 'hand over' to the Approved Social Worker/Approved Mental Health Practitioner or psychiatrist (where the patient/client is being held under Section 136). Once the patient has been assessed and admission is deemed the way forward, a psychiatric nurse will be required to wait with the patient, if there is likely to be a long delay for bed availability. (Note that the patient may be in contact with a Community Psychiatric Nurse (CPN); it may be of value to make contact with the CPN for information.)

Please be aware that the 2007 Act has replaced the title of Approved Social Worker with that of Approved Mental Health Practitioner; this opens up the function to professionals other than social workers. Social Service authorities are to retain responsibility for approving professionals, and training courses will be subject to statutory regulation, as well as approval by the General Social Care Council (England) or Care Council for Wales. The Mental Health Act (1983/2007) was designed to protect the individual from potential abuses to their freedom, while protecting the public and the patient from any consequences of the mental illness. Approved Mental Health Practitioners/Approved Social Workers, GPs and specialist approved doctors (psychiatrists) are usually involved in assessing the patient for a Section Order. This multi-disciplinary approach to invoking the Section Order is designed to protect the patient from unnecessary admission and removal of human rights.

There are a variety of Sections within the Act that may be used to secure a patient's admission; see Box 8.4.

Box 8.4 Sections of the Mental Health Act (2007) that are relevant to the ambulance clinician

Section 2 (Admission for assessment)
Admission for up to a period of 28 days. Two doctors make recommendation for admission, one of whom must be approved. Assessment from both doctors within a period of five days of each other.

Section 3 (Admission for treatment)
Admission for up to a period of six months, renewable for periods of up to one year at a time for severe mental illness/impairment /disorder, which requires treatment in hospital.

Section 4 (Admission for assessment in an emergency)
Admission for a period of up to 72 hours (the patient can be placed under Sections 2 or 3 after examination) for urgent assessment.

Section 131 (Informal admission)
The patient voluntarily agrees to be admitted, but can change her mind and refuse. There is no time limit.

Section 135 (Place of safety order – private)
Admission for a period of up to 72 hours. A person suffering from mental illness can be removed from a private dwelling to a place of safety, for assessment. The patient should not be removed directly to hospital under Section 135 unless an Approved Mental Health Practitioner/Approved Social Worker or GP has attended.

Section 136 (Place of safety order – public)
Admission for a period of up to 72 hours. A person suffering from a mental illness can be removed from a public place to a place of safety (usually a police station or possibly a hospital) by a police office or an Approved Mental Health Practitioner/ Approved Social Worker.

> Under the 2007 Mental Health Act, both Sections 135 and 136 have been amended to allow transfers between places of safety, within the 72-hour detention period. Transfer during the 72-hour detention period was not allowed under the 1983 Mental Health Act. This is an area where ambulance clinicians may be asked to provide safe transfer of patients under either of these two sections.

For further reading see JRCALC (2006); Department of Health (2007).

Conclusion

This chapter has hopefully provided the reader with an understanding of some of the psychological problems that a child, young person and adult can face. We may agree to define psychological abnormalities as patterns of functioning that are:

- dysfunctional (interfering with the person's ability to conduct daily activities in a constructive way);
- deviant (different, extreme, unusual, perhaps even bizarre);
- distressful (unpleasant and upsetting for the sufferer and significant others);
- dangerous (to oneself or to others, hostile and careless)

(Comer 2004)

However, we should be clear that these criteria are often vague and subjective and not all sufferers will show all behaviours. It is also important to mention that, despite popular misconceptions, most sufferers with anxiety, depression, and even bizarre thinking pose no immediate danger to themselves or to others. However, as an ambulance clinician/healthcare professional you should at all times make an assessment of your personal safety when approaching an upset, disorientated, agitated or threatening patient/client. If you think you are at considerable risk you may need to call the police who are suitably trained for these situations (JRCALC 2006).

As an ambulance clinician you will encounter sufferers of psychological problems in your working life. It is essential that you have an awareness of the theoretical underpinnings to your practice in order that you can assess and care for these sufferers holistically and competently. It is important that your approach to these patients/clients should be calm and you should take your time to communicate during assessment. Do not rush, because a distressed or agitated person may react negatively to being hurried, and always be honest about what is going to happen.

 Stop and think – Below is a useful mnemonic (GASPIPES), in terms of thinking through the assessment of a patient/client's mental state. Ask yourself whether the patient/client is experiencing any of the following:

G uilt and self-reproach
A ppetite is disturbed
S leep disturbance, suffering insomnia

P aying attention to your questions or not, orientation to time, place and person
I nterest in things lacking, such as football, music etc.
P sychomotor disturbance – slow, agitated, pacing, mood, hallucinations and belief expressed
E nergy – loss, tired, slow
S uicidal – expressed thoughts

Chapter key points

• The ambulance clinician requires an awareness of the signs and symptoms of mental ill health and guidelines given by the Mental Health Act (1983/2007) and Trust policy in order to assess a patient's condition correctly and instigate appropriate treatment or obtain specialist assistance (the capacity of the patient/client to consent must be assessed).

• Ambulance clinicians should be aware of their personal safety at all times.

References and suggested reading

Achenbach, T. (2003) *Assess adaptive and maladaptive functioning. Achenbach System of Empirically Based Assessment (ASEBA)*. London: Harcourt Press.

Alzheimer's Society (2007) Dementia UK. A report into the prevalence and cost of dementia prepared by the Personal Social Services Research Unit (PSSRU) at the London School of Economics and the Institute of Psychiatry at King's College, London, for the Alzheimer's Society. London: Alzheimer's Society.

American Psychiatric Association (2000) *Diagnostic and Statistical Manual of Mental Disorders*. DSMIV. Philadelphia, PA: American Psychiatric Association.

Appleby, L. (1999) *Safer Services: National Confidential Inquiry into Suicide and Homicide by People with Mental Illness*. London: Department of Health.

Audit Commission (1999) *Children in Mind. Child and Adolescent Mental Health Service*. London: Audit Commission.

Barton, R. (2007) Use of medication in children with psychiatric disorders, *Community Practitioner*, 80(11): 42–3.

Beck, A.T. (1967) *Depression: Clinical, Experimental and Theoretical Aspects*. New York: Harper Row.

Beck, A.T. and Friedman, A. (1990) *Cognitive Therapy of Personality Disorders*. New York: Guilford.

Berger, K.S. (2003) *The Developing Person through Childhood and Adolescence*. New York: Worth Publishers.

Bird, L. (1999) *The Fundamental Facts*. London: Mental Health Foundation.

Bird, L. and Faulkner, A. (2000) *Suicide and Self-Harm*. London: Mental Health Foundation.

Bowlby, J. (1969) *Attachment and Loss. Volume I: Attachment*. London: Hogarth Press.

Caroline, N.L. (2007) *Emergency Care in the Streets*, 6th edn. London: Bartlett and Jones/British Paramedic Association.

Charlton, J., Kelly S., Dunnell, K., Evans, B. and Jenkins, R. (1994) *The Prevention of Suicide*. London: HMSO.

Comer, R.J. (2004) *Abnormal Psychology*, 5th edn. New York: Worth.

Craig, T.K.J., Hodson, S., Woodward, S. and Richardson, S. (1996) *Off to a Bad Start: A Longitudinal Study of Homeless Young People in London*. London: Mental Health Foundation.

Craig, T.K.L. and Hodson, S. (1998) Homeless youth in London: 1. Childhood antecedants and psychiatric disorder, *Psychological Medicine*, 28: 1379–88.

Davison, G.C. and Neale, J.M. (1997) *Abnormal Psychology*, 7th edn. New York: John Wiley & Sons.

De Silva, P. and Rachman, S. J. (1998) *Obsessive-Compulsive Disorder: The Facts*. Oxford: Oxford University Press.

DfES (Department for Education and Skills) (2003) *National Service Framework for Children, Young People and Maternity Services*. London: DfES.

DoH (Department of Health) (1999) *Saving Lives: Our Healthier Nation*. London: HMSO.

DoH (1983) *Mental Health Act*. London: DoH.

DoH (1999) *National Service Framework for Mental Health: Modern Standards and Service Models*. London: DoH.

DoH (2005) *Mental Capacity Act*. London: DoH.

DoH (2007) *Mental Health Act*. London: DoH.

De Silva, P. and Rackman, S. (1998) *Obsessive-Compulsive Disorder: The Facts*, 2nd edn. Buckingham: Open University Press.

Eysenck, H.J. (2000) *Psychology: A Student's Handbook*. Hove: Psychology Press.

Gelder, M., Gath, D., Mayou, R. and Cowen, P. (1996) *Oxford Textbook of Psychiatry*, 3rd edn. Oxford: Oxford University Press.

Goldberg, D. and Huxley, P. (1992) *Common Mental Disorders: A Bio-social Model*. Oxford: Routledge.

Gorenstein, E.E. and Comer, R.J. (2002) *Case Studies in Abnormal Psychology*. New York: Worth.

Gotlib, I.H. and Hamen, C.L. (1997) *Psychological Aspects of Depression. Towards a Cognitive-Interpersonal Integration*. Chichester: Wiley and Sons.

Green, H., McGinnity, A. and Meltzer, H. (2004) *Mental Health of Children and Young People in Great Britain*. London: Office for National Statistics.

Hale, A. (1997) ABC of mental health: anxiety, *British Medical Journal*, 314, 28 June: 1886–9.

Hale, A. (1997) ABC of mental health: depression, *British Medical Journal*, 315, 5 July: 43–6.

Hammen, C. (1997) *Depression*. Hove: Psychology Press.

Hasnie, B. (2007) Anti-social adolescents conduct disorder: a review, *Community Practitioner*, 80 (7): 38–40.

Hawton, K. and Fagg, J. (1998) Suicide, and other causes of death, following attempted suicide, *British Journal of Psychiatry*, 152: 359–66.

Healy, D. (1998) Gloomy days and sunshine pills, *Openmind*, 90, March/April.

Hewstone, M., Fincham, F.D. and Foster, J. (2005) *Psychology*. Oxford: BPS and Blackwell.

Hill, K. (1995) *The Long Sleep: Young People and Suicide*. London: Virago.

JRCALC (Joint Royal Colleges Ambulance Liaison Committee) (2006) *UK Ambulance Service Clinical Practice Guidelines*. London. JRCALC/Ambulance Service Association (ASA).

Kalat, J.W. (1995) *Biological Psychology*, 5th edn. New York: Brookes Cole Publishing Company.

Kapur, N., Turnbull, P., Hawton, K., Simkin, S., Sutton, L., Machway-Jones, K. *et al.* (2005) Self-poisoning suicides in England: a multicentre study, *An International Journal of Medicine*, 98 (8): 589–97.

Lane, A. (1997) Postnatal depression and elation among mothers and their partners: prevalence and predictors, *British Journal of Psychiatry*, 171: 550–3.

Lazarus, R.S. and Folkman, S. (1984) *Stress, Appraisal, and Coping*. New York: Springer.

McAllister, M., Geedy, D., Moyle, W. and Farrugia, C. (2002) Nurses' attitudes towards clients who self-harm, *Journal of Advanced Nursing*, 40(5): 578–86.

McLaughlin, C. (2007) *Suicide: Understanding, Caring and Therapeutic Response*. London: Wiley.

Mental Health Foundation (1997) *Suicide and Deliberate Self-Harm. The Fundamental Facts*. Bristol: Mental Health Foundation. www.mhf.org.uk/Brief001.htm. (Accessed 9 August 2007.)

Office for National Statistics (2000) *Psychiatric Morbidity among Adults Living in Private Households in Great Britain*. London: Office for National Statistics.

Office for National Statistics (2003) *Health Statistics Quarterly. Trends in the Mortality of Young Adults Aged 15–44 in England and Wales, 1961 to 2001*. London: Office for National Statistics.

Office for National Statistics (2006a) *Surveys of Psychiatric Morbidity among Adults in Great Britain*. London: Office for National Statistics.

Office for National Statistics (2006b) *Better or Worse: A Longitudinal Study of the Mental Health of Adults Living in Private Households in Great Britain*. London: Office for National Statistics.

Pelkonen, M. and Marttunen, M. (2003) Child and adolescent suicide: epidemiology, risk factors, and approaches to prevention, *Pediatric Drugs*, 5 (4): 243–63.

Pembroke, L., Smith, A. and the National Self-harm Network (1998) *Minimising the Damage from Self-Harm: The Guide for Friends, Relatives and Advocates going with a Person who Self-Harms to an Accident and Emergency Department*. London: National Self-harm Network.

Rachman, S. and de Silva, P. (1996) *Panic Disorder: The Facts*. Buckingham: Oxford Paperbacks.

Roy, A. (1996) Asian wives driven to suicide, *Daily Telegraph*, 22 April.

Royal College of Psychiatrists (2007) www.rcpsych.ac.uk/pressparliament/mentalhealthact 2007.aspx. (Accessed 8 August 2007.)

Samaritans (2004) *Information Resource Pack 2004*. Ewell: Samaritans.

Seligman, M.E.P. (1973a) *Authentic Happiness*. New York: Random House.

Seligman, M.E.P. (1973b) Fall into helplessness, *Psychology Today*, June: 96–103.

Selikowitz, M. (1998) *Down's Syndrome: The Facts*, 2nd edn. Buckingham: OU Press.

Shneidman, E.S. (1985) *Definition of Suicide*. New York: Wiley.

Smith, P.K., Cowie, H. and Blades, M. (2003) *Understanding Children's Development*. Oxford: Blackwell.

Stewart, G. (2000) *Men's Mental Health* Factsheet. London: MIND.

Stewart, G. (2005) *Men's Mental Health. Factsheet*. London: MIND.

Tsuang, M. and Faraone, S. (1998) *Schizophrenia: The Facts*. Buckingham: Open University Press.

Zimbardo, P., McDermott, M., Jansz, J. and Metaal, N. (1995) *Psychology: A European Text*. London: Harper Collins.

Useful websites

Department for children, school and families: www.dfes.gov.uk

Department of Health: www.dh.gov.uk

Intellectual Disability website: This site was developed as a collaboration between the Down's Syndrome Association and the Division of Mental Health at St George's, University of

London, with financial support from GUS Charitable Trust and the Department of Health. This is a web-based learning resource for medical and healthcare students and practitioners, launched at the Houses of Parliament in 2002. It provides up-to-date information about the health needs of people with intellectual disabilities: www. intellectualdisability.info/home

The charity Mental Health: www.mentalhealth.org.uk

National Association for Mental Health: www.mind.org.uk

National Statistics online, provided by the Office of National Statistics, government departments and devolved administrations: www.statistics.gov.uk

Office of the Children's Commissioner http://www.11million.org.uk. This is the media, publications and general information centre for the 11 million led by the Children's Commissioner. The web address is derived from the following statement: 'The 11 million children and young people in England have a voice' (Children's Commissioner for England, Professor Sir Albert Aynsley-Green).

Office of Public Sector information: www.opsi.gov.uk

Royal College of Psychiatrists: www.rcpsychs.ac.uk

Samaritans: www.samaritans.org/know/pdf/InforResourcePack2004web.pdf

Young Minds. http://www.youngminds.org.uk. A national charity committed to improving the mental health of all children and young people through giving advice, training and campaigning.

9

Safeguarding children
Jackie Whitnell

Topics covered:

- Introduction
- Why is this relevant?
- Organizations, legislation and reform
- 'Tools of the trade' (frameworks/guidance)
- What is child abuse and neglect?
- Why does abuse and neglect happen?
- Indicators of abuse and neglect
- Child protection and children with special needs/disability
- Domestic abuse and children
- Conclusion
- Chapter key points
- References, suggested reading and useful websites

Introduction

The prime focus of this chapter for ambulance clinicians and healthcare professionals is to heighten awareness around safeguarding children and provide a basic understanding of what is meant by the term 'child in need' and child protection. This chapter commences with frameworks for guidance for professionals and then continues with discussion around causes, indicators and effects of child abuse, children with special needs and/or disability and consideration for children living with domestic abuse. Hopefully this chapter will provide information for the ambulance clinician and healthcare professional to make relevant links between theory and practice.

Why is this relevant?

Stop and think – Before reading on do you know of any important policies, frameworks or guidance that aid the healthcare profession in safeguarding children? Jot them down.

In 2003, the government, acknowledging that safeguarding children is everyone's responsibility, set out an ambitious plan: a new approach to children's policy, *Every Child Matters* (ECM) (DfES 2003) – a reform of children's services. The goal was, and remains, to help all children fulfil their potential and for professionals to identify and provide services for those children *in need*. It is essential that healthcare professionals, which includes ambulance clinicians, should pay attention to the needs of all children, not just those who are already considered children *in need* or those children that have suffered abuse or neglect. Service provision may be required for children with learning disabilities, sensory impairment, children that are living in poverty and/or social exclusion, children with a disability and children with a parent or parents with learning disabilities. Services may also be required for children with parent(s) who are suffering with mental illness, drug and alcohol misuse, children who are being poorly parented or are in an environment where domestic violence occurs. At all times the ambulance clinician is in the position to prevent a child from possibly being harmed by providing relevant information to other agencies and healthcare professionals who take over the care of the child.

The intention of the new policy is that children's services will be more preventive than reactive. Thus policy is requiring a change in practice by organizations and individual healthcare professionals. However, it is still paramount that the well-established world of child protection continues for children who are suffering or are at risk of suffering from significant harm (Munro 2007). The essence of the ECM (DfES 2003) is that all children should have a chance to fulfil their potential. Children and young people informed the government's working party that they considered the following five outcomes to be essential in achieving their potential:

- Be healthy
- Stay safe
- Enjoy and achieve
- Make a positive contribution
- Achieve economic well-being

There are already, and have been historically, important organizations and documents that guide professional inter-agency/multi-agency cooperative working, including *Every Child Matters* (DfES 2003), some of which will be discussed below.

Organizations, legislation and reform

1887 saw the inception of the National Society for the Prevention of Cruelty to Children (NSPCC). This came about from the condemnation of parental violence towards children; this organization has made substantial inroads in safeguarding children from harm (www.nspcc.org.uk). 1989 saw the introduction of the Children Act. This document set out a new balance between the State and the family in terms of prevention of child abuse and neglect. 1989 also brought about the United Nations Convention for the Rights of the Child (UNCRC), to which all four countries of the UK are signatories. The UNCRC provides the framework for legislation and practice and asserts that children and young people's needs are important and unique. The framework maintains a child-centred focus and helps to identify concerns about possible maltreatment. It also reflects the need to consult with children and young people on all aspects of their daily lives. In relation to this, it is considered that the child is an individual with rights and not the property of adults (HM Government 1991).

The Children Act (1989) was revised in 2004. This latest legislation is not to be compared with the 1989 Act and does not supersede it, but it does introduce many reforms to the system, many of which have their origins in the recommendations of the Victoria Climbie inquiry (Laming 2003) and *Every Child Matters* (DfES 2003). Some of the reforms include:

- establishing Children's Commissioners for all four countries in the UK (Sections 1–9). The posts are independent from government, and were created to ensure that the views and interests of children are represented across the UK;
- providing modernized ways of working in the assessment and support of children in need;
- establishing a database of children (Section 12) to enable healthcare professionals to 'track' children across agencies in order to safeguard them from potential harm;
- bringing together social care and education under one umbrella;
- local authorities to appoint 'Directors of Children's Services' (Section 18); and
- establishing 'Local Safeguarding Children Boards' (Sections 13–16) in each local authority area.

'Tools of the trade' (frameworks/guidance)

2006 saw the revised version of *Working Together to Safeguard Children* (DfES 2006c). This revised version provides core guidance on how agencies should cooperate and work together in safeguarding and promoting the welfare of children and how to respond to concerns that a child may be at risk of significant harm. This core guidance relates to the revised Children Act (DoH 2004b).

The *Common Assessment Framework* (CAF) (DfES 2006b) aligns to the five outcomes of ECM (DfES 2003). This ecological framework has much to offer children who are potentially vulnerable and/or are *in need*, as well as those affected by child abuse, neglect and domestic violence. An ecological framework described by

Belsky (1993) reflects a four-level approach:

- ontogenic development (the parent's developmental background and experiences);
- the microsystem (the interaction of individuals within the family);
- the exosystem (the immediate social environment within which the family functions);
- the macrosystem (the broader structural factors, such as cultural attitudes to drugs).

The way in which these systems interact with each other is extremely valuable when assessing parenting skills and the potential for child maltreatment. The CAF (DfES 2006b) helps practitioners to identify both strengths and needs within families.

A *child in need* is a child who is unlikely to achieve or maintain a reasonable standard of health or development without appropriate provision of services from a local authority (DoH 1989). Early assessment and intervention is essential to ensure that children, their mothers, fathers and siblings receive supportive intervention from the local authorities, in the hope that they may not have to go through the statutory service. This tool can be used by many professionals and requires further multi-professional education on assessment of *children in need* and child protection. In terms of education and training this will heighten awareness of ambulance clinicians and other healthcare professionals and improve service provision towards early intervention.

A further tool ('**graded care profile**'), specifically designed for the assessment and management of neglect, provides practitioners with a comprehensive tool that aids assessment of parenting capacity and the means to negotiate targets for improving parenting and thus outcomes for the child. This tool is drawn from the work of Maslow, allowing the practitioner to *rate* parenting in relation to safety, love and esteem. The tool provides objective measurements of the balance of risk and protective factors in the parent and child dyad. This tool was trialled in 1997 and the general consensus was that the tool can identify good parenting in spite of poverty and hardship; however, even though this is a good tool it has to be said that it is not overly used in all practices. Assessment can be complex and it can be difficult to engage with some families, especially those that are suffering disadvantage. If parent/s are struggling to provide 'good enough' care they may be suffering from low self-esteem and may well believe that they cannot change anything and the healthcare professional cannot help them to do so.

If on assessment there is concern that a child may be at risk of significant harm, a thorough assessment under the *Framework for Assessment of Children in Need and their Families* (DoH 2000) may be required. This triadic assessment considers three factors which includes the child's developmental needs, family and environmental factors, and parenting capacity (see Figure 9.1).

By undertaking this initial formal assessment, the local authority can then ascertain whether:

- the child is a *child in need* and the local authority has a duty to help (a *child in need* is defined in Section 17 (10) of the Children Act 1989) and/or;

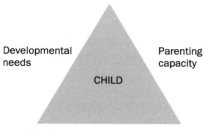

Developmental needs

Parenting capacity

CHILD

Family and environmental factors

Figure 9.1 Based on the Framework for Assessment
Source: DoH (2000)

- there is reasonable cause to suspect that the child is suffering, or is likely to suffer, significant harm (Section 47 of the Children Act 1989). This section sets out that the local authority has a statutory duty to investigate whenever it has reasonable cause to suspect that a child lives, or is found to live, in their area.

As discussed, there are many tools used in order to safeguard children. These are extremely useful in terms of improving practice, identifying needs and encouraging systematic thinking about a family, as well as being an aid to the decision-making process in the progress of child abuse cases. However, tools alone are not enough; they need to predict along with reason. As professionals, we need to reason our judgements based on analysis and intuition. Analytic reasoning is generally formal, explicit and based on logic, each step spelled out in a rigorous process. In contrast, intuition is largely unconscious, quick and guided by the individual's understanding of people – how they feel, how they behave and how they act. You could argue that this is instinctual *gut feeling*. It helps if healthcare professionals use both analytical reasoning *and* intuition when engaging with children and families, in order to gain their cooperation and collect information.

Ambulance clinicians will use their reasoning powers in terms of analysis and logic, but also trust their intuitive instincts in terms of making an assessment in safeguarding children. Reasoning can have errors; it is difficult not to make judgements and it needs to be based on knowledge, non-biased and anti-discriminative practice. As an ambulance clinician or healthcare professional you will have personal views and values about what is or is not acceptable parenting, whether you are a parent or not. Healthcare professionals should be open at all times to other people's thoughts and concerns, as we are all capable of making misjudgements. The Cleveland Enquiry is a case in point. This was an investigation into the incorrect diagnosis by a healthcare professional that many children had been sexually abused. This caused much distress to the families concerned at the time and for a long time after the event (DoH 1988).

Link to chapter 4, pages 34–7 for an explanation of more theoretical perspectives and exploration of how to try and work in an anti-discriminatory manner.

The patient report form (PRF) is a document subject to audit used to relay valuable information to other healthcare professions. As an ambulance clinician you will transfer children during the course of your practice. It is likely that you will see children in their home environment and it is possible that you may observe a home environment that you feel is unacceptable and unsafe. This is a difficult dilemma. You may want to mention your observation to the receiving staff and/or make a comment on your patient report form if you have concerns regarding the safety of the child. If you have concerns for a child's safety you would not only communicate your information verbally to other healthcare professionals; you would also follow the ambulance service and the Trust's operational guidelines and complete the **Safeguarding children report form** (DoH 2003; JRCALC 2006, appendix 2.3).

Stop and think – When viewing a home environment ask yourself: is it unsafe or just untidy? Is it 'chaotic' or just lived in?

There may be situations in which you have to separate your personal values from your professional role and this can be difficult (e.g. in observing an environment that did not meet with your own standards). In this instance you should seek the advice of your crew mate/rapid response staff or control staff to ascertain their professional standpoint. Many times in your working practice you may have to be certain of your professional role, not personal judgement, to ensure that families are judged against society's standards around what is acceptable. Ultimately, the judgement is about what is or is not potentially harmful for the child.

Link to Chapter 16 to explore the role of the HPC in providing guidance to paramedics, and the professionals' responsibilities in such difficult circumstances.

Further assistance in safeguarding children is provided by recent statutory reconfiguration of the Area Child Protection Committee (ACPC) to the **Local Safeguarding Children Board** (LSCB) in England and Wales. Under the auspices of the Children Act (DoH 2004b) the LSCB has a wider remit. The LSCB details local guidance procedures; it is required to draw up local policies and procedures, covering thresholds for intervention, training, recruitment of staff who work with children and investigation of allegations about staff working with children. The Board is made up of key people who can provide valuable guidance for healthcare professionals and provide contact details. They are responsible for coordinating efforts across local agencies to safeguard children and for looking into issues arising from child deaths (Beckett 2007).

In England the *National Service Framework*, (DfES 2004b) core standard 5 states that: 'All agencies work to prevent children suffering harm and to promote their welfare, provide them with the services they require to address their identified needs and safeguard children who are being or who are likely to be harmed.' A number of markers of good practice are identified:

- Local development of safeguarding policies, procedures and practices, including for those who recruit and manage staff e.g. Independent Safeguarding Authority (ISA, previously the Independent Barring Board), is set up to help prevent unsuitable people from working with vulnerable people and to make the workforce safer for children and vulnerable adults. The ISA will be developing a register of people who should not work with children or vulnerable adults. This decision has come about from the recommendations (No.19) of the report made by Sir Michael Bichard from the Soham/Bichard (2004a) inquiry which states that 'New arrangements should be introduced requiring those who wish to work with children or vulnerable adults to be registered. The register would confirm that there is no known reason why an individual should not work with these client groups.' There will also be a list of people where there are reasons why they should not work with children and vulnerable adults.

- Actively involving children, young people and families in assessment processes and ensuring accessibility of universal services e.g. health, education and housing.

- Particular note is made of the vulnerability of children with special needs and/or disability (Hobbs *et al.* 1999; NWGCPD 2003; Sobley 2006).

- Need for training and support of all staff that have roles and responsibilities in safeguarding children within their working day.

- Standards 5 and 7 to be achieved by 2014.

Between the 1989 Children Act and the 2004 revised Act the Laming Report (Laming 2003) was written, based on the Victoria Climbie case. Victoria (born 2 November 1991 on the Ivory Coast) was in the privately arranged foster care of her aunt Marie Therese Kouao who had taken Victoria to France and then to London to live. Victoria's aunt was to obtain a better education and greater opportunities for Victoria's future. However, Victoria suffered for 11 months while in London at the hands of her aunt and her aunt's new partner Carl Manning from multiple abuse. After her death at age 8 years and 3 months on 25 February 2000, she was found to have suffered from hypothermia and 128 separate injuries. Victoria was known to four social service departments, one NSPCC centre, three housing authorities, two police child protection teams and had been seen at two hospitals, as well as being in the care of other health professionals such as health visitors. The Laming Report (2003) has many recommendations but essentially they are that:

- confidentiality must be maintained to protect the child (but not to the detriment of the child);
- thorough assessment of children is vital;
- there should be appropriate adequate communication between agencies at all times; and
- thorough factual information must be documented.

The Laming Report (2003) and recommendations are laid down in the hope that we do not see a repeat of Victoria's case. As an ambulance clinician, again it is fundamental to be reminded that you are in an extremely valuable and important position to refer appropriately on to other health professionals should you be at all concerned for a child considered *in need* or who may have other child protection issues.

This part of the chapter has summarized the 'tools of the trade' used for *children in need* and for children in need of protection, in order to provide the reader with an awareness of the current policy and guidance. We will now consider what constitutes child abuse and neglect, looking particularly at signs and symptoms, to raise the awareness of ambulance clinicians and healthcare professionals. This section will also look at safeguarding children with special needs and consider children living within a home in which there is domestic abuse.

What is child abuse and neglect?

In simple terms, child abuse and neglect can be defined as treating a child harmfully and immorally. There are many definitions, both local and global, which are broad and specific, that can lead to confusion. Definitions change over time and are socially constructed. For examples see:

- National Commission of Enquiry into the Prevention of Child Abuse (1996)
- World Health Organisation – www.who.int
- DfES (2006c) (See Box 9.1)

Box 9.1 Definitions of child maltreatment/categories of abuse

1.27 *Abuse and neglect* are forms of maltreatment of a child. Somebody may abuse or neglect a child by inflicting harm, or by failing to act to prevent harm. Children may be abused in a family or an institutional or community setting; by those known to them or, more rarely, by a stranger. They may be abused by an adult or adults or another child or children.

1.28 *Physical abuse* may involve hitting, shaking, throwing, poisoning, burning or scalding, drowning, suffocating, or otherwise causing physical harm to a child. Physical harm may also be caused when a parent or carer fabricates the symptoms of, or deliberately induces illness in, a child (Royal College of Paediatrics and Child Health (RCPCH 2002) for more on fabricated/induced illness (FII).

1.29   *Emotional abuse* is the persistent emotional maltreatment of a child such as to cause severe and persistent adverse effects on the child's emotional development. It may involve conveying to children that they are worthless or unloved, inadequate, or valued only in so far as they meet the needs of another person. It may feature age or developmentally inappropriate expectations being imposed on children. These may include interactions that are beyond the child's developmental capability, as well as overprotection and limitation of exploration and learning, or preventing the child participating in normal social interaction. It may involve seeing or hearing the ill treatment of another. It may involve causing children frequently to feel frightened or in danger, or the exploitation or corruption of children. Some level of emotional abuse is involved in all types of maltreatment of a child though it may occur alone.

1.30   *Sexual abuse* involves forcing or enticing a child or young person to take part in sexual activities, including prostitution, whether or not the child is aware of what is happening. The activities may involve physical contact, including penetrative (e.g. rape, buggery or oral sex) or non-penetrative acts. They may include non-contact activities such as involving children in looking at, or in the production of pornographic material or watching sexual activities, or encouraging children to behave in sexually inappropriate ways.

1.31   *Neglect* is the persistent failure to meet a child's basic and/or psychological needs, likely to result in the serious impairment of the child's health or development. Neglect may occur during pregnancy as a result of maternal substance abuse. Once a child is born, neglect may involve a parent or carer failing to provide adequate food or clothing, shelter including exclusion from home or abandonment, failing to protect a child from physical or emotional harm or danger, failure to ensure adequate supervision including the use of inadequate care takers, or the failure to ensure access to appropriate medical care or treatment. It may also include neglect of, or unresponsiveness to, a child's basic emotional needs.

(DfES 2006c: 8)

Box 9.1 highlights the overall definition of child abuse and neglect and the individual categories of maltreatment that are used in a child protection conference and applies at present to the categories in which children are placed on the child protection ('at risk') register. The child protection conference involves a multi-agency approach to safeguarding the child and includes the parent/s if they wish to attend. The conference determines whether or not the child is at risk of continuing harm and, if so, establishes a core group to develop and implement a formal *child protection plan*. At the time of writing the use of a 'child protection register' is due to be discontinued; however, if a child or young person has a *child protection plan* this should be identifiable on the database of social care records.

Definitions are a useful benchmark but they are not always easy to apply to practice and decision making. Lawrence (2004) argues that there is no substantive definition of the term 'child abuse or neglect'. Child maltreatment is a complex construct that has been (and may well always be) interpreted in many different ways. As mentioned before, definitions and tools are useful but should be used alongside consideration for facts, reasoning, awareness of cultural differences, diversity of parenting, actual evidence, social context and actual harm. Box 9.2 highlights facts and statistics from different sources.

Box 9.2 Child abuse/neglect facts and statistics

14.8 million children (0–19 years) in the UK, three million children in need (ONS 2004)

The UK is widely recognized to have one of the highest rates of child poverty in the industrialized world, 1:4 children living in poverty (Jose 2005). However, the number has decreased in recent years (HM Government 2006)

26,4000 children on the at risk register (DfES 2006a) Risk of neglect = 43 per cent increase on previous years; risk of emotional abuse = 21 per cent; physical abuse 16 per cent and sexual abuse 9 per cent; the remaining 11 per cent were 'mixed' categories

Every week in England and Wales one–two children under 16 years of age are killed at the hands of another person (ONS 2006)

Two-thirds of these deaths are in children aged 5 years or less and in 60 per cent of all cases parents are the principal suspects (ONS 2006)

Infants under 1 year of age are most at risk of being killed and in these cases mothers and fathers are equally likely to kill the infant (ONS 2006)

Why does abuse and neglect happen?

There is much research based on this question. Research has provided the healthcare professional with valuable information about the factors that could lead to the risk of abuse. This research has produced useful predictive factors which can help towards identification of the potential for child abuse (Marziali *et al.* 2003). However, these factors do not mean causation *per se*. Understanding risk factors can help the healthcare professional predict children at risk and children in need, this being one of the key strategies within ECM (DfES 2003) policy and the intention of the CAF tool of assessment (DfES 2006b). However, professionals need to be aware that a link or predictive factor, for example poverty, does not necessarily mean neglect is likely to occur – this would be a weak predictive factor. A strong predictive factor, however, would be the unusual bruises on a child's buttocks when in fact the child wears nappies 24 hours a day; this would indeed trigger suspicion of abuse.

Let us look further at why abuse happens, in terms of theories of causation or links. Abuse is considered to be multi-factorial due to the differences in family structures and cultures within society and the interplay of many differing aspects of family life. Among the many theories are those from psychology, socio-cultural, biological and a mixture of all three. In terms of attachment theory, Bowlby (1979) argues that if parents had insecure attachments in their childhood to their prime carer this could be a risk factor in the way that they care for their own children. Insecure attachment could link to a person possibly having low self-esteem and maybe an anxious personality. This could have consequences for their child's emotional development and possibly put the child at risk of abuse or neglect (Bowlby 1979; Howe 2005).

> Link to Chapter 7 for more theory and information on attachment theory.

Psychologically, parents may suffer from social isolation due to the inability to attach to others. They may have a low tolerance level and unrealistic expectations of their child/children. They may find their child's behaviour difficult to manage and feel incompetent as a parent, leading them to be angry towards their child/ren. Bandura (1971) argued that in terms of social learning theory, children will model themselves on others, especially those close to them e.g. parents. If they experience violence and abuse they may think it normal practice and use it to express their own emotions. This indicates a cycle of abuse; however, research has only provided links, not causal relations, to this theory (Powell 2007).

> Link to Chapter 7 for discussion around social learning theory.

There are situations where abuse occurs and it is considered to be the fault of parent psychopathology. The parent may have suffered or be suffering from mental illness, personality disorder or learning disabilities which have manifest in some form of violence towards the child through their own depression, or neglect of the child maybe due to ignorance and/or poor parenting (Falkov 1996; Sanders *et al.* 1999; Dale *et al.* 2002; Sinclair and Bullock 2002). It has been argued over the last decade that child health services and mental health services should work more closely together. Other socio-cultural issues that have been considered as risk factors are poor housing, social class, poverty, social exclusion and stress (Sanders *et al.* 1999). Jose (2005) debates the definitions of poverty and its links with child abuse and neglect, arguing that one in four children are living in poverty. She states that healthcare professionals have a duty both to recognize poverty and its effects on children and to provide help and support to disadvantaged families. There are many predictive factors that healthcare professionals and/or ambulance clinicians should be aware of in order that they attempt to safeguard the child (Sidebotham 2003). In the ECM (DfES 2003) policy there is an attempt at a multi-dimensional approach to help reduce poverty, improve housing and education, improve parenting skills and provide support for families. The ECM considers there is no one theory but a collection of socio-cultural, psychological factors that can be the reason why children are in need or, indeed, why child abuse and neglect occurs, and all situations must be considered.

Link to Chapters 6 and 11 for more theoretical perspectives concerning psychology and sociology, which will inform the reader.

It is important that as an ambulance clinician/healthcare professional you have an awareness of what constitutes possible child abuse and be able to recognize some potential signs of Non-accidental Injury (NAI). It is also essential that you are aware of local Trust policies and operational procedures in the event that you need to report a child that you suspect is at risk. Consequently, you should be familiar with your service's operational guidelines (JRCALC 2006).

Indicators of abuse and neglect

When assessing the possibility of NAI you should use judgements regarding whether the injury and the story given is appropriate for the age of the child in terms of development. (Does the picture fit the story?) An understanding of normal development is essential in determining what a child would ordinarily be able to do at differing ages. There are children (those with learning disability) that may be not developing according to the 'norm' and that should be taken into account when assessing a child; stages of development can vary. Children may crawl or walk at different ages. However, in terms of injuries that may or may not be accidental, there are injuries that would be extremely difficult to obtain at certain ages and it is in your best interest and the child's for you to have knowledge of these; for example, a non-mobile baby with bruises to legs or feet would raise concern. Healthy babies do not bruise themselves when thrashing about in play or against cot sides. However, a toddler who is running around may well have obtained bruises to temple or shins. This knowledge is useful in determining potential abuse, but when assessing an injured child you should keep an open mind and consider your findings carefully, based on knowledge and the carer's story, and ascertain whether the explanation is credible. If you are at all concerned always document and report your findings on the patient report form and if necessary the safeguarding children report form when handing over the child's care to other healthcare professionals.

Link to Chapter 7 for child development and an understanding of a child's development at certain ages.

Examples of abuse indicators may be:

- any injury in a non-mobile baby;
- frequent accidents in unlikely places, e.g. the buttocks, trunk, inner thighs;
- soft tissue injuries, bruises under clothing e.g. nappies;
- bruises the same age on both sides of the body or of varying ages;
- small deep burns in unlikely places or repeated burns and scalds (not to be confused with old chicken pox scars, scabies or impetigo);
- poor state of clothing, cleanliness and/or nutrition (unkempt appearance);
- late reporting of the injury or delay in seeking help (JRCALC 2006).

Physical abuse

Injuries that would raise concern in a non-mobile baby:

- Bruising on ears, face, neck, trunk and buttocks (round small bruise on each cheek indicates mouth being held tight, maybe to force bottle feed).
- Petechial spots (tiny blood spots under the skin) which vanish quickly may indicate attempted smothering.
- A torn frenulum (behind the upper lip) and/or bleeding from the mouth.
- Fractures: these are uncommon in babies; bones are bendy and do not easily break.
- Shaking of baby may show finger bruising on the chest. Other brain injuries would not be seen by ambulance clinicians but indicators might be, continued high-pitched scream or low consciousness when neurologically assessed.
- Burns and scalds are only common over six months of age by accident. Burns are only found on palms of hands, not on backs of hands. Scald by pulling hot liquids would be found as splash marks.
- Other causes for concern may be recurrent A & E attendances, failure to thrive and induced or fabricated illness (RCPCH 2002).

Injuries that would raise concern in a mobile baby or toddler:

- Bruising is common for mobile babies and toddlers; they are usually on the front of the body as children are likely to fall forward.
- They do not bruise on both sides of body or around a curved surface.

Types of bruising include:

- striped – indicates imprint of fingers;
- tramline – indicates the use of belt or stick;
- Part or all of circle – indicates bite marks;
- Round small – indicates force of grip.

Old and new bruises will be different colours depending on age; always observe the colours of bruises if there are more than one. You may want to draw them (actual size) on your safeguarding report form if you are concerned.

- Abusive burns are often deep and small and may show outline of object whereas accidental burns will not, because reflexively, the child would pull away.
- Cigarette burns are round and deep and have a red flare around a flat brown crust.
- Scalds – again, splash marks indicate accidents and in toddlers are very common; however, a scald that is bilateral, for example both feet to a specific line, would indicate dunking a child in boiling water feet first.
- Fractures generally are uncommon. A fracture that would be cause for concern is one which goes around the bone due to a twisting force; this is often considered an NAI (spiral fracture).

There has been much controversy around the issue of giving a child a 'smack' or 'spank' as punishment. To reason and negotiate with a child who is being totally unruly is the optimum management, but many parents from time to time resort to more physical tactics to try and control and discipline their child (Howe 2005). Many cultures accept such practices as normal, appropriate and understandable. However, there is a point along the physical disciplinary continuum where chastisement (e.g. a tap on the back of a hand) can tip into unreasonable aggression or physical abuse (e.g. a slap that leaves a mark) and even greater unreasonable punishment (e.g. slap on the face) (DoH 2004b: Section 58). This year (2007) the government, following a review of legislation, rejected a ban on smacking children. The review found that smacking 'is becoming a less commonly used form of discipline' and the majority of parents said there should be no outright ban. It was considered by the junior children's minister Kevin Brennan that 'The police have discretion to deal with cases as they consider appropriate, taking into account factors including the evidence available, the public interest and the best interests of the child.' Consequently, the government will retain the law on smacking under Section 58 of the Children Act 2004 (DoH 2004b). The Children's Commissioner for England, Sir Al Aynsley-Green, was among critics including children's charities that called for a ban on smacking. He said he was 'disappointed' at the government's decision. He argues: 'This is a missed opportunity to protect children from violence in the home and that young people should have the same rights to protection under the law on common assault as that given to adults.' It would appear that government and parents consider there to be no good reason why children are the only people in the UK who can still be hit lawfully in the home. Are we sending out confusing messages to parents and children about the acceptable use of violence across society? (For more information on this issue see the website www.communitycare.co.uk, listed at the end of this chapter.)

Stop and think – Have you heard people say 'It did me no harm'? This statement almost legitimizes the use of unreasonable aggression.

When making an assessment of injury it may be useful to remember that older children and young people are likely to give an accurate account if the injury is accidental. However, if the injury was non-accidental the child will often provide a story that is not making *sense* or does not fit the injury. This may occur, especially if they have been told what to say by the perpetrator. Self-harm injuries and overdosing may be a cry for help, indicating abuse or exploitation. As an ambulance clinician you will transfer babies, toddlers, children and young people with injuries. It is essential, in order to safeguard children, that you have a foundation of knowledge of the indicators of physical abuse. The injuries are likely to be easier to detect than that of other abuse e.g. emotional, sexual and neglect. This chapter will continue with discussion around the other categories of abuse and neglect.

Emotional abuse

This form of abuse can be difficult to recognize; a child can appear well cared for and live in a comfortable environment. Emotional abuse will occur alongside all other categories of abuse and neglect as it is impossible to remove the emotion of what is happening to the child. It is important that as a healthcare professional you are aware of factors that may indicate a child is suffering from emotional abuse:

- Ignoring – if the parent does not show any love or attention and continually ignores the child.
- Terrorizing – if the parent has unrealistic expectations of the child.
- Rejecting – if the child is blamed for things that go wrong or is *persistently* told they may be unloved or sent away.
- Isolating – if the child is continually given the impression that the parents are disappointed in them.
- Corrupting – the child is used for labour or involved in unacceptable acts.
- Verbally assaulting – persistently told the parent/carer/sibling wished the child was never born; that they are hated or stupid.
- Over-controlling – parents who are obsessive about cleanliness, tidiness, over-loving, not allowing child's own expression.

Children can be at risk of emotional abuse because of situations in which they live, such as parent with mental illness, home with domestic violence occurring, or parent with alcohol or drug misuse problem. It is important that you note the parent's attitude towards the child and consider: is it unfeeling; is there bad handling; is the parent over-anxious? If you detect such behaviour, it would be important to inform the healthcare professional to whom you hand the child over and document your findings on your patient report/safeguarding children report form.

Sexual abuse

Commonly the abuser is known to the child; abuse can occur by other children and/or siblings as well as an adult. Mostly abuse occurs by male abusers, but occasionally women will abuse children, or aid and abet the abuse. It is always difficult for society to accept that the very person/people with whom the child's care is entrusted and who is responsible for their child's protection, behind locked doors, can be the abuser. The notion of 'stranger danger' is inaccurate, but it is much easier for us as a society to fear the stranger rather than those who are trusted within and by the family (Wilczynski 1997).

Sexual abuse is difficult to detect as there are few physical signs; indicators are often emotional and behavioural factors. Below are some factors that may indicate sexual abuse is occurring:

Physical factors:

- Vaginal soreness, bleeding, discharge.
- Urinary tract infection (UTI) and/or vaginal infection, bruising, bite marks.
- Sexual transmitted disease (STD).
- Pregnancy.
- Soiling, constipation.

Emotional and behavioural factors:

- Inappropriate knowledge or sexual approaches for age and stage of development.
- Fear at bath or bedtime.
- Drug, alcohol abuse, self-harm.
- Frozen watchfulness, stares into space, does not engage with you.
- Unnatural compliance.
- Fear of medical help.
- Withdrawal of physical contact or play.
- Clothes that cover all parts of the body at an inappropriate time of year (summer day).

Neglect

Defined as 'needs not being met'. It could be difficult to detect, until failure to thrive is occurring. Consider the following factors when you assess the child, parents and home environment:

- Neglect of physical care such as warmth, nourishment, safety; hygiene poor/ unkempt look; may have rashes on body or nappy area; insect bite marks (tiny pinhead); scabies marks that can resemble cigarette burns.
- Failure to encourage development, impairment of growth, intellect.
- Poor attachment, unfeeling, ignoring.
- Unhappy child, miserable, continually crying, hiding in corners, aggressive or timid.
- Unusual behaviours e.g. rocking, head banging.

Take the Family Held Record (Red Book) if it is available to the hospital for assessment of previous percentile charts of weight, height and head circumference (if previously completed).

Impact

As an ambulance clinician you are in an extremely valuable position to identify the possible abuse factors and in some situations you may be the professional that has a valuable piece of information (a piece of a puzzle) that is essential to safeguarding a child. You may be the person to whom the child or parent discloses.

In all cases of abuse, the child is suffering, and will not have his/her needs met. It is imperative that, at all times, safeguarding children is everyone's responsibility (DfES 2003). It is important to recognize and respond to concerns about a child in need. Your concerns should be shared with other professionals. There is a child protection adviser in most Trusts available to offer guidance; at the very least you would report your findings on the patient report form/safeguarding report form and hand over you concerns verbally to the receiver. Child protection is an emotive issue and it may be that you would seek some personal support or discussion for yourself. This is essential in some cases.

Child protection and children with special needs/disability

Children in this group have particular needs and may be more vulnerable to abuse. Sullivan and Knutson (2000) found that this group of children are three times more likely to experience emotional abuse than other children. Some may demonstrate challenging behaviour which can be difficult to manage at times. They may live in a stressful home environment. Some of the many factors that can cause stress for these children are:

- Language – be conscious that English may not be the first language of the child.
- Post-traumatic stress disorder (PTSD) – be conscious that you may well be caring for people that are seeking asylum and/or are refugees.
- Physical disability – be sensitive to people with disabilities; children/young people; ascertain what they are capable of doing for themselves.
- Learning disability – you will care for children and people with a learning disability and they may not fully understand what you are asking of them. You may need props, symbols and so on to get your point across.

Link to Chapter 7 for more detail about atypical behaviour.

Domestic abuse and children

Domestic abuse is very much in the media spotlight and society's concern about it has risen markedly in recent years for two main reasons:

1   it often co-exists with child abuse; and
2   its occurrence has a detrimental impact on the child/children in the family (Humphreys and Mullender 2005).

Domestic abuse is involved in two-thirds of the cases presented in child protection conferences (Munro 2007) and the Metropolitan Police Domestic Violence Strategy (Metropolitan Police 2001) was put together to help those suffering from domestic abuse. It is important to raise the healthcare professional's awareness, and the information here will provide an understanding of this issue.

The box below highlights different definitions of abuse. You will note that one is based on the seeing or hearing of domestic violence; the other provides an explanation of what constitutes domestic violence.

Definitions of domestic violence

Impairment suffered from seeing or hearing ill treatment of another (Home Office 2002).

Any incident of threatening behaviour, violence or abuse (psychological, physical, sexual, financial or emotional) between adults who are, or have been, intimate partners or family members, regardless of gender or sexuality (DoH 2005).

Most children are aware if a parent is being abused and up to 86 per cent of domestic abuse incidents occur when the children are in the same or an adjoining room (DoH 2005). Children and young people (including unborn children) who are at risk of exposure to domestic abuse need to be identified, protected and supported. Exposure to domestic abuse can lead to symptoms not unlike those suffered from post-traumatic stress disorder, for example emotional numbing, increased arousal, depression and aggressive behaviour (Parkinson and Humphreys 1998). Children are often affected by domestic abuse and show behavioural and emotional disturbance. Research highlights external behaviour as aggression and being antisocial, and internal behaviour as anxiety or depression. Some children are more resilient than others in dealing with adversity and some parents will deny that the child is aware of the abuse but most children have some knowledge of what is going on and suffer some form of reaction (National Commission 1996; Calder *et al.* 2004). Children are exposed through observation and/or getting involved to protect their mother (DfES 2003). Research suggests that 45–70 per cent of children suffer physical abuse when living with domestic abuse (Howe 2005). Children living with domestic abuse are at risk of significant harm through direct physical or sexual violence. There is also evidence of domestic abuse associated with neglect and psychological mal-treatment plus the emotionally damaging effects of hearing or witnessing the abuse and from the consequences and the ability of the non-abusing parent to parent effec-tively (McGuigan and Pratt 2001; Powell 2007).

Ambulance clinicians and healthcare professionals need to be more aware of the critical links between domestic abuse and child abuse and be better placed to enquire and respond to disclosures, at the same time as ensuring their own safety and that of sufferers and their children. The Local Government Association (LGA) (2006) is concerned with integrating services for domestic abuse with the children's agenda and this forms part of the LSCB's role.

Violence between adult partners occurs in all social classes, all ethnic groups and cultures, all age groups, in those with disabilities as well as the able-bodied, and in both homosexual and heterosexual relationships. Women are usually the most fre-quent victims. The dominant pattern is of violence and abuse of women. However, there are minority groups, i.e. same-sex relationships and elder abuse of men and women. Domestic abuse has profound consequences in the lives of individuals, chil-dren, families and communities. Social cultural explanation often blames the media, suggesting it legitimizes violence. There are strong links between domestic abuse and other risk factors for child maltreatment, including parental substance misuse and mental health needs (Amnesty International 2006). There is heightened incidence of substance misuse by victims, in order to manage the domestic abuse, and an increase in mental health issues and health problems affecting the women victims e.g. depres-sion, anxiety, low self-esteem and social isolation (Howe 2005). This can affect the parenting of children.

Conclusion

All healthcare professionals in contact with children should have some form of 'safe-guarding children', child protection and domestic abuse awareness in order that they are able to identify concerns in a child's health and development. Children and fam-ilies come from diverse situations and different cultures which can make safeguarding children more complex. It is imperative that the ambulance clinician and healthcare professional is able to provide an appropriate response to a concern, and know who to report and refer the concern to, so that it does not escalate into a more serious problem. It may be that English is not the child or family's first language and an interpreter may be required in the follow-up when you hand over the child's care. The ambulance clinician will need to seek out and record the views of the child (if pos-sible). It is imperative that you hand over your assessment and complete the patient report form and, if appropriate, the safeguarding children report form in full, in order that the receiver of the child can make the necessary referral and obtain the appropri-ate help. As an ambulance clinician or healthcare professional you are in a prime position and it is important that you do the following:

- Observe the interaction between the child and carer. Is it warm, caring?
- Detect tensions between child and carer/s.
- Consider any inappropriate behaviour and report it to the person taking over

your care and document your findings. Your assessment could form a piece of a puzzle.

- Have an understanding of child protection issues and domestic abuse.
- Consider what are the needs of the child.
- Think about whether the parents/carers are responding appropriately to the child's needs/care and showing compassion.
- Consider whether the child is being adequately safeguarded from harm in the home environment.
- Know where to take your concerns; who to report them to.
- **It is vitally important, and in fact essential, that at all times you have a kind and reassuring approach towards the child. Never lie about what is going to happen. The child must feel she can trust you (JRCALC 2006).**
- **Any allegation of abuse by a child is an important indicator and should be taken seriously and investigated, even if it turns out to be fabrication.**
- **Always take the Family Held Record (Red Book), if it is available, to the hospital for completion by staff.**

Chapter key points

- The ambulance clinician requires an understanding of the policy surrounding safeguarding children in order to fulfil professional responsibility.
- Ambulance clinicians should have an awareness of the signs of child abuse and neglect, which is vital to enable them to recognize potentially dangerous situations for children and to act for, and protect, vulnerable children.

References and suggested reading

Amnesty International (2006) *Making the Grade?* London: Amnesty International UK.

Bandura, A. (1971) *Social Learning Theory.* Morristown, NJ: General Learning.

Beckett, C. (2007) *Child Protection: An Introduction.* London: Sage Publications.

Belsky, J. (1993) Etiology of child maltreatment: a developmental–ecological analysis, *Psychological Bulletin,* 114 (3): 413–34.

Bowlby, J. (1979) *The Making and Breaking of Affectional Bonds.* London Tavistock.

Calder, M., Gordon, H. and Howarth, E. (2004) *Children Living with Domestic Violence: Towards a Framework for Assessment and Intervention.* Lyme Regis: Russell House Publishing.

Commission on Families and the Well-being of Children (2005) *Families and the State.* www.nfpi.org.uk/dagta/research/docs/family-commission-exec-summary-31.doc.

Corby, B. (2006) *Child Abuse: Towards a Knowledge Base,* 3rd edn. Maidenhead: Open University Press.

Dale, P., Green, R. and Fellows, R. (2002) *What Really Happened? Child Protection Case Management of Infants with Serious Injuries and Discrepant Parental Explanations.* London: NSPCC.

DfES (Department for Education and Skills) (2003) *Every Child Matters.* London: DfES.

DfES (2004a) *Every Child Matters: Change for Children.* London: DfES.

DfES (2004b) *National Service Framework for Children, Young People and Maternity Services*. London: DfES.

DfES (2005) *Common Core of Skills and Knowledge for the Children's Workforce*. London: DfES.

DfES (2006a) *Referrals, Assessments and Children and Young People on Child Protection Registers, England – Year Ending 31 March 2006*. London: The Stationery Office.

DfES (2006b) *Common Assessment Framework*. London: DfES.

DfES (2006c) *Working Together to Safeguard Children*. London: DfES.

DoH (Department of Health) (1988) *Report of the Inquiry into Child Abuse in Cleveland, 1987*. London: HMSO.

DoH (1989) *Introduction to the Children Act*. London: HMSO.

DoH (1995) *Child Protection: Messages from Research*. London: The Stationery Office.

DoH (2000) *Framework for the Assessment of Children in Need and their Families*. London: The Stationery Office.

DoH (2003) *What To Do If You're Worried a Child Is Being Abused*. London: The Stationery Office.

DoH (2004a) *Bichard Inquiry*. London: The Stationery Office.

DoH (2004b) *The Children Act*. London: The Stationery Office.

DoH (2005) *Responding to Domestic Abuse: A Handbook for Health Professionals*. London: Department of Health.

Falkov, A. (1996) *Study of Working Together Part 8 Reports: Fatal Child Abuse and Parental Psychiatric Disorder – An Analysis of 100 ACPC Case Reviews Conducted Under the Terms of Part 8 of Working Together under the Children Act 1989: A Guide to Arrangements for Inter-agency Co-operation for the Protection of Children from Abuse*. London: Department of Health.

HM Government (1991) *The United Nations Convention on the Right of the Child*. London: TSO.

HM Government (2006) *Reaching Out: An Action Plan on Social Exclusion*. London: Cabinet Office.

Hobbs, C., Hanks, H. and Wynne, J. (1999) *Child Abuse and Neglect: A Clinician's Handbook*. London: Churchill Livingstone.

Home Office (2002) *Adoption and Children Act*. London: TSO.

Howe, D. (2005) *Child Abuse and Neglect*. New York: Palgrave Macmillan.

Humphreys, C. and Mullender, A. (2005) *Children and Domestic Violence: A Research Overview of the Impact on Children*. Dartington: Research in Practice, www.rip.org.uk.

Humphreys, C. and Stanley, N. (2006) *Domestic Violence and Child Protection: Directions for Good Practice*. London: Jessica Kingsley.

Joint Royal Colleges Ambulance Liaison Committee (2006) *UK Ambulance Service Clinical Practice Guidelines*. London: JRCALC/Ambulance Service Association (ASA).

Jose, N. (2005) Child poverty: is it child abuse?, *Paediatric Nursing*, 17 (8): 20–3.

Laming, Lord H. (2003) *The Victoria Climbie Inquiry*. London: The Stationery Office.

Lawrence, A. (2004) *Principles of Child Protection: Management and Practice*. Maidenhead: Open University Press.

LGA (Local Government Association) (2006) *Vision for Services for Children and Young People Affected by Domestic Violence*. London: Local Government Association.

McGuigan, W. and Pratt, C. (2001) The predictive impact of domestic violence on three types of child maltreatment, *Child Abuse and Neglect*, 25: 869–83.

Marziali, E., Damianakis, T. and Trocme, N. (2003) Nature and consequences of personality problems in maltreating care givers, *Families in Society*, 530–8.

Metropolitan Police (2001) *Enough is Enough: Domestic Violence Strategy*. London: Metropolitan Police.

Munro, E. (2007) *Child Protection*. London: Sage Publications.

National Commission of Enquiry into the Prevention of Child Abuse (1996) *Childhood Matters*, Vol. 1. London: HMSO.

NSPCC Inform (2006) *Child Homicides*. www.nspcc.org.uk/inform/onlineresources/statistics/KeyCPstats. (Accessed 30 November 2007.)

NWGCPD (National Working Group on Child Protection and Disability) (2003) *It Doesn't Happen to Disabled Children*. London: NSPCC.

Office of the Children's Commissioner (2006) *Annual Report 2005/06*. London: The Stationery Office.

Office for National Statistics (2002) *Social Focus in Brief: Children*. London: ONS.

Office for National Statistics (2004) *The Health of Children and Young People*. London: ONS.

Office for National Statistics (2006) *Mortality Statistics: Childhood, Infant and Perinatal* (Series, DH3 No 37). London: ONS.

Parkinson, P. and Humphreys, C. (1998) Children who witness domestic violence: the implications for child protection, *Child and Family Law Quarterly*, 10: 147–59.

Powell, C. (2007) *Safeguarding Children and Young People: A Guide for Nurses and Midwives*. Maidenhead: Open University Press/McGraw-Hill.

RCPCH (Royal College of Paediatrics and Child Health) (2002) *Fabricated or Induced Illness by Carers*. London: Royal College of Paediatrics and Child Health.

Sanders, R., Colton, M. and Roberts, S. (1999) Child Abuse Fatalities and Cases of Extreme Concern: Lessons from Reviews, *Child Abuse and Neglect*, 23 (3): 257–68.

Sidebotham, P. (2003) 'Red skies, risk factors, and early indicators', *Families in Society*: 530–8l.

Sinclair, R. and Bullock, R. (2002) *Learning from Past Experience: A Review of Serious Case Reviews*. London: DoH.

Sobley, D. (2006) Special cases, not double standards, please, *Child Rights Information Network Newsletter*, 19: 30–3.

Stevenson, O. (2007) *Neglected Children and Their Families*. Oxford: Blackwell.

Sullivan, P. and Knutson, J. (2000) Maltreatment and disabilities: a population-based epidemiological study, *Child Abuse and Neglect*, 28: 267–7.

Tutt, R. (2007) *Every Child Included*. London: Paul Chapman.

Wall, K. (2006) *Special Needs and Early Years: A Practitioner's Guide*. London: Paul Chapman.

Wilczynski, A. (1997) *Child Homicide*. London: Greenwich Medical Media.

Wilson, K. and James, A. (2002) *The Child Protection Handbook*. London: Bailliere Tindall.

Useful websites

Childline – a charity to provide assistance and help for people affected by abuse: www.childline.org.uk

Department for Education and Skills (DfES) main website: www.dfes.gov.uk; see also www.standards.dfes.gov.uk

Department of Health (DoH/DH) main website: www.dh.gov.uk

Every Child Matters – government site about the reform of children's service: www.everychildmatters.gov.uk

Families in Society – the journal of contemporary social services. A forum for addressing the interests, activities and concerns of professionals, management supervision, education, research, policy and planning: www.familiesinsociety.org

The Hideout – support for children and young people living with domestic violence: www.thehideout.org.uk

Joseph Rowntree Foundation: www.jrf.org.uk

NSPCC – National Society for Prevention of Cruelty to Children, a valuable resource for professionals: www.nspcc.org.uk/kidszone

Women's Aid – site for women and children living with violence: www.womensaid.org.uk

World Health Organization: www.who.int

10

Sociology: an introduction
Amanda Blaber

Topics covered:

- Introduction
- Why is this relevant?
- Characteristics of sociology
- Introduction to classical sociologists
- Conclusion
- Chapter key points
- References and suggested reading

Introduction

This chapter will introduce the classical sociologists and their theories to the reader. The chapter contains a modern-day example and relates sociologists' principles to the example, in order that the reader appreciates the salience of the theories in twenty-first century Britain.

Why is this relevant?

All professionals working within the NHS have contact with members of Britain's society. So why do ambulance clinicians require an understanding of sociology and its key concepts? Ambulance clinicians and other healthcare community workers are unique in the sense that they see people in their own social world, i.e. their homes, with families, friends and in their part of society (location). Hospital-based workers do not see people functioning in their own environments because being hospitalized brings them into the hospital organization, with its own culture. If ambulance clinicians have a wider understanding of why people talk and act, respond to illness and operate within society in the way that they do, clinicians may be able to adjust their own behaviour accordingly, when dealing with patients. This would obviously improve the experience for both clinician and patient and may enhance the overall quality of care provided.

Link to Chapter 4, pages 34–9, to appreciate the importance of practising in an anti-discriminatory manner at all times.

Characteristics of sociology

Many people find the study of sociology frustrating because it does not have concrete answers. The study of anatomy and physiology is very different: you know it or you don't and there is little ambiguity about the facts. Successful sociology requires students to open their minds and eyes, be curious, ask questions about the world around them and to think about and discuss their own ideas. There are many key theorists who have done just that, have become eminent in their field and have created concepts that can be applied to our social world today. This is perhaps a good starting point for students who have not studied sociology before, as it provides concepts to explore and discussion in relation to the twenty-first century. Every action has a reaction; sociology may assist you in experiencing positive rather than negative reactions on a daily basis. If nothing else, it should make you curious to try and understand (a little more) about people and the society in which we all live. Students may also learn something about themselves.

Introduction to classical sociologists

Durkheim

There are three classical sociologists whose work originates from the eighteenth century but does have relevance today. As Bilton *et al.* (2002) explain, Durkheim explores the nature of societies. Durkheim developed the concept of 'social solidarity' to explain the various ways in which societies can be integrated. Durkheim also explained other types of solidarity such as mechanical solidarity, where individuals identify with each other, usually because they have similar lives. Durkheim applied this to pre-modern societies, with respect to clans and tribes. Regarding modern societies, Durkheim identified that no individual or section of society could function without engaging in interaction with others; he termed this organic solidarity. Durkheim states that a complete society is reliant on the close interrelationship between individuals and sections of society (Bilton *et al.* 2002).

Stop and think – As an individual, how many sections of society are you reliant upon on a daily basis?

As an ambulance clinician responding to a person trapped, after a road traffic accident, how would you know about the accident in order to get dispatched?

How would you get there without the mechanical support from your ambulance Trust? Would the equipment you carry be working? Would the roads be open and negotiable if roadworks and traffic lights were not maintained? Could you treat the person trapped without the help of the other emergency services . . . and so on? This should give you an idea of what Durkheim was trying to illustrate with the concept of organic society.

Bilton *et al.* (2002) state that where individuals act independently of commonly recognized norms of behaviour or social standards, Durkheim used the term 'anomie' to explain their behaviour. Durkheim believed societies were at greater risk of social disintegration because of the growth of individualism and self-importance. With this comes the increase of divergence of experience and values for members of society.

Stop and think – In your daily working lives you meet people who have chosen to act outside the norms of social standards or behaviour. Think of some examples. This is the concept of anomie that Durkheim proposed.

Durkheim's final concept suggests that sociologists should 'treat social facts as things'. An example of this concept is best explained by the reality of suicide, as explained by Bilton *et al.* (2002). Suicide was a subject that Durkheim studied in terms of social causes, rather than explaining it in terms of individual or psychological factors. Bilton *et al.* (2002: 6) ask: 'Why are young men, more than any other social group, at risk of taking their own lives?' Recent statistics for the UK confirm that since 1997 the highest rates of suicide have been in men aged 15 to 44 years. It has not always been the case in the UK; in the early 1990s the highest suicide rate was in men aged 75+. The rate of men committing suicide (17.5 suicides per 100,000 population) has been consistently higher than women (six suicides per 100,000 population) throughout the 1991–2005 period (ONS 2006). Durkheim believed suicide was due to social factors more than anything else.

Stop and think – In your experience of suicide, is this the case?

Durkheim put forward his theory of functionalism and stated that society works as a social system and is not just made up of social facts. The ways we think and live are established in a culture and can be called institutionalized behaviour and beliefs, in sociological terms. Bilton *et al.* (2002) explain that the integration, solidarity and balance of a society are maintained by institutions such as the family, political system, education system, legal system, each performing their functions properly and interdependently. For students who prefer human biology, think of our society as a human body: there are organs that perform necessary functions to keep a human healthy.

This is a functionalist principle. Bilton *et al.* (2002) state that the main criticism of this concept is that it omits the role people play in each of society's functioning systems.

> Link to Chapter 11 to read about the areas of our lives and how these factors are linked.

Biography

Emile Durkheim (1858–1917). War played a large part in Durkheim's life; the 1870–71 defeat of France by Prussia occurred in his early years and the First World War (1914–18) in his latter years. Durkheim was brought up as an Orthodox Jew. His father was a rabbi and this was a path Emile was expected to follow, until his conversion to Catholicism, then agnosticism in his youth. Durkheim was very much an academic; he went to school in Paris, where his interest in social and political philosophy developed. He went on to teach philosophy, preferring to debate in terms of theoretical principles rather than enter the political arena. Durkheim spent a year in Germany, impressed by advances in social science and psychology. In 1887 Durkheim worked at the University of Bordeaux; it was during this period that his major works were written. Durkheim's reputation led him to the Sorbonne, Paris, as professor of education and social science in 1902 (Marsh and Keating 2006).

As with Durkheim (1964), Marx (cited in Coser 1977) was interested by and examined the dynamics of societies and the changes that take place in societies over time, in particular to explain the evolution of capitalism and how this, he believed, would eventually lead to a communist system. Marx, unlike Durkheim's functionalism, is concerned with exploring conflict in society. Marx wrote a great deal and there are various interpretations of his many works (Marsh and Keating 2006). One of Marx's concepts, mode of production, describes ways in which production of goods, needed for individuals to survive and prosper, was organized in society. Marx argued that in a capitalist society the motivation for the production of goods is for profit (Bilton *et al.* 2002). The prevalence of 'mad cow' disease/bovine spongiform encephalitis (BSE) within the last 10 to 20 years, Marx would argue, is a direct consequence of using the remains of animals as farm feed, as a cheaper option, thus increasing the farmer's profit margin. In addition to 'mad cow disease'/BSE the recent outbreaks of foot and mouth disease also demonstrate the point that the quest for profit can have catastrophic consequences.

 Stop and think – Review the evolution of BSE or 'mad cow disease'. This is able to transfer to humans and is termed new variant CJD (Creutzfeld-Jakob disease). It has been proven that the cause was the use of cheaper feed given to cows; this included animal by-products being processed into the feed for naturally herbivorous animals, in the name of profit (Bilton *et al.* 2002).

Read the following press extract. Could this happen again? Is profit more of a driver than the health and safety of society?

Health fears grow as mountains of meat are smuggled into the UK

The amount of illegal meat entering Britain may be far higher than previously thought, increasing concerns about contamination of the food chain.

New figures disclosed by the Department for the Environment, Food and Rural Affairs (Defra) show the amount seized by customs and local authority environmental health teams has risen by almost 600 per cent in the last six years. Defra minister Ben Bradshaw said 104 tons of illegal meat was seized last year, compared with 18.6 tons in 2001.

Previously the government's Veterinary Laboratories Agency had estimated that an average 12,000 tons of meat enters Britain illegally each year, carried in by passengers travelling through ferry terminals and airports, via mail and hidden in containers on sea tankers. But the sixfold rise in seizures suggests the true figure could be dramatically higher.

Defra has increased funding to tackle the problem, amid concerns that infected produce could enter the food chain. The move was prompted by concerns that the foot-and-mouth outbreak of 2001, which cost the taxpayer £8bn, was a result of contaminated meat imported in pigswill. At Heathrow airport alone there are now four teams of customs officials dedicated to detecting illegal meat.

The illegal meat trade in Britain takes many forms. Much of it is smuggled in from Eastern Europe and China. Some of it is in the form of 'smokies', the blowtorched carcasses of sheep or goats which are a West African delicacy. Around 2 per cent of the illegal imports is bushmeat – exotic meat such as zebra, ant-eater or monkey – which is highly prized among Afro-Caribbean communities.

Concerns have increased amid revelations the European Union is considering allowing the remains of animals to be used as farm feed for the first time since the BSE crisis.

(Doward 2007)

Marx

Biography

Karl Marx (1818–83). Born in the Rhineland of Germany, at university his political ideas became more radical. He had numerous influences in his life as a result of living in Paris, working as a journalist and meeting numerous people. In Paris, Marx studied economics and was introduced to the ideas of socialism and communism. Marx briefly revisited Germany during the revolution, moved to London and was exiled there in 1849. From then on Marx spent his time trying to build a workers' party and analysing capitalism, as he believed political power is closely linked to economic power (Marsh and Keating 2006).

Marx used class analysis as one of his central themes. Marx saw power as being unequally distributed across societies and believed that economic power is the basis for other forms of power.

Stop and think – Look at the BSE example and the fact that cheaper meat would be most likely to be bought by people in lower social classes and was also at a higher risk of BSE due to cheaper feed being given to these animals. Is what Marx was implying in his concept, developed in the eighteenth century, still applicable today?

The concept of alienation has a strict definition in Marxism but this has been used in broader terms than Marx first intended. Bilton *et al.* (2002:10) state that Marx believes alienation 'describes the ways in which individual workers become separated from the products of their labour, from each other and from other classes through the organisation of production in specifically capitalist ways'. A broader view of Marxist alienation could be applied to the BSE crisis.

Stop and think – Do you know where the meat you eat originates from? In light of the BSE episode do you trust the farming industry? Marx would suggest that you have a sense of distrust, which may explain the 'boom' in local farmers' markets.

Marsh and Keating (2006) suggests that two distinct forms of Marxism have developed since Marx's death: structural Marxism concerned with class exploitation and the importance of economics and humanist Marxism, focused upon the alienation of the human spirit due to capitalism.

Weber

Biography

Max Weber (1864–1920). Born in Germany; throughout his life saw massive changes in Germany's industrial status in the world. Towards the end of Weber's life Germany first challenged Britain as a leading industrial power. Weber worked as an academic in economics and political economy. This work was intermittent, as Weber's bouts of depression and nervous breakdown at the time of his father's death prohibited him from continuously working (Marsh and Keating 2006).

Definition of modernity

Becoming a modern society.

Definition of rationalism

A way of thinking, regulated by reason rather than intuition or emotion.

Weber's work expresses his own fears and anxieties about modernity, which he believed was irreversible. Weber believed that an individual's needs would not be fulfilled by the material gain, increased power and economic dependence that modernity brings. One of Weber's central themes was that rules, regulations and laws naturally accompany capitalist modernity and that society would become dependant on this organized structure. Weber believed 'rational–legal' authority characterized modern society. He believed this is based upon impersonal rules that have been rationally formalized and organized without emotion or intuition and have created bureaucracy. Weber introduced the concept of social action and called on sociologists to examine the consequences of individuals; these may not always be intended or anticipated. Weber calls the individuals 'social actors'. In terms of the BSE crisis, Bilton *et al.* (2002) suggest that Weber would encourage sociologists to examine the meanings and intentions of all parties, farmers, government officials, consumers, the media and others to examine the motivation, in addition to the consequences of their actions.

 Stop and think – How many times have you heard 'Not my job'; 'More than my job's worth'?

With respect to the BSE/'mad cow' disease crisis, all involved had their own motives. One of the 'social actors' being the consumer, the motives of the majority of consumers may have been wanting cheaper meat, which they thought would meet certain government standards. When the disease developed, despite standard setting, the media exposed the BSE crisis. As a consequence, those who could afford to do so bought more expensive meat, chose not to eat meat, or only bought meat from local sources they felt they could trust. This goes some way to explain Weber's sociological perspectives.

Conclusion

The classical theorists' work still has resonance in the twenty-first century. Other sociologists have developed their thinking and theories based upon the classical sociologists' concepts; the following chapters will aim to introduce the student to some of these more contemporary concepts. There are key areas of our lives that have an influence on 'who we are': our social class, our family, our education and our work are examples. Some of these areas will be examined in terms of sociological theory, in order that students can link theory to their own lives and the lives of patients.

Chapter key points

- The work of the classical sociologists still has resonance today.
- It is possible to relate sociological theory to modern examples.
- Our own lives and lives of others can be explored and understood through sociological theory.
- Sociology should encourage us to question and discover our own self and explore the world around us.

References and suggested reading

Bilton, T., Bonnett, K., Jones, P., Lawson, T., Skinner, D., Stanworth, M. and Webster, A. (2002) *Introductory Sociology*, 4th edn. Basingstoke: Palgrave Macmillan.

Coser, L.A. (1977) *Masters of Sociological Thought. Ideas in Historical and Social Context.* New York: Harcourt Brace.

Doward, J. (2007) *Health fears grow as mountains of meat are smuggled into the UK*, Observer, 10 June. www.environment.guardian.co.uk/print/0,,330001740–121570,00.html. (Accessed 2 July 2007.)

Durkheim, E. (1964) *The Rules of the Sociological Method.* New York: Free Press.

Marsh, I. and Keating, I. (2006) *Sociology. Making Sense of Society*, 3rd edn. London: Pearson Education Limited.

Office for National Statistics, General Register Office for Scotland, Northern Ireland Statistics and Research Agency (2006) *Suicides. Rate in UK Men Continues to Fall.* London: ONS.

11

Social factors
Amanda Blaber

Topics covered:

- Introduction
- Why is this relevant?
- Socialization
- Social stratification
- Gender and sexuality
- Families and family life
- Culture
- Race
- Religion
- Education
- Age
- Work
- The mass media
- Crime
- Conclusion
- Chapter key points
- References, suggested reading and useful websites

Introduction

This chapter will introduce you to the main factors that affect all of our lives and how we function within society. All of the factors discussed will seem familiar, such as families, work and age.

Why is this relevant?

As well as introducing some new concepts/theorists, the chapter is intended to invite you to question areas of your life that you may take for granted and have grown up with. Although brief (in comparison with sociology texts), the chapter hopes to raise the student's awareness of sociology and how it can assist us in understanding ourselves and others. There are references to ambulance clinician work and readers are invited to explore their thoughts on certain areas of social life. Many areas will require further reading in order to avoid just 'skimming the surface' of a subject; suggested reading has been included.

Socialization

Definition of norm

Socially accepted 'correct' or 'proper' form of behaviour. 'Norms either prescribe given types of behaviour or forbid them' (Bilton *et al.* 2002: 16).

Definition of values

Ideals and beliefs regarded as important by a society or social group (Bilton *et al.* 2002: 16).

Biography

Charles Cooley (1864–1929) was a United States sociologist who developed his theory of symbolic interactionism in the 1920s and 1930s. Another writer in this area is George Mead, who linked social behaviour with social psychology.

Socialization is an important sociological term and is perhaps an appropriate starting point for students to begin to question why they are who they are. This process commences at birth. Marsh and Keating (2006: 263) define socialization as 'the term given to the process by which we learn the norms, values and roles approved by our society'.

The initial stages of a child's development are primarily with parents and members of the family and are face-to-face. As a child grows up, other influences, such as school and friends, are involved in a child's development; this is when formal social rules are predominantly learnt. Cooley (1909, cited in Ritzer 1996) describes the initial face-to-face socialization as being undertaken by a primary group and the latter stages as secondary group socialization. It is when children enter other social institutions, such as school, that they realize they form part of a 'larger picture' and are, perhaps for the first time, judged by society's rules and standards. This is described as Cooley's 'primary group' theory. Another of Cooley's concepts (1902, cited in Kornblum 1997) was the 'looking glass self', where we judge ourselves as we imagine others see us. This concept has three steps:

1   We imagine how we present ourselves to others; for example, are we smart, caring, tall, funny?

2   Then we interpret how people react to us; for instance, do they see us as we see ourselves, or do they see something else?

3   We then use interpretations of others' reactions to us, to develop our sense of self. If we sense that people disagree with our perception of our self, then our 'self-concept' will diminish; we may change our behaviour. If we think we agree with others, self-concept will become stronger.

Cooley's approach is described as symbolic interaction.

Stop and think about yourself. Who would you say constituted your primary group during your socialization? Who constituted your secondary group? Does this process ever stop? Has your pre-hospital education socialized you in a different way?

Link to Chapter 7 for more reading about the theories of development.

During socialization with both primary and secondary groups, an individual forms an identity. Sociologists suggest that identity formation is a combination of the physical, the personal and the social. During the process of growing up the individual does not take on all influences, but reflects, negotiates and incorporates (or rejects) them.

Biography

Erving Goffman (1922–82) considered all individuals to 'act' for their audiences in everyday life. His approach is interactionist. Goffman argued that our behaviour follows patterns and that individuals follow a set of instructions that influence and determine behaviour (Goffman 1963).

Our interactions between ourselves and the world we live in help establish our identity. Sociologists, such as Cooley (1902, cited in Kornblum 1997 and 1909, cited in Ritzer 1996), Mead ([1934] 1967) and Goffman (1963) believe our identities are subject to change and not assigned at birth. Most of us have a variety of identities that we adopt according to our varying roles in society, for example, parent, colleague, paramedic, student (Goffman 1963; Cohen 1994).

Stop and think – How many different identities do you have? How closely are these associated with the roles you have within society?

Marsh and Keating (2006) suggest that as our socialization with the secondary group increases we will influence others' views of us by using dress and language. For example, consider the influence (either positively or negatively) of your uniform. In order to challenge your own first impressions you should take time to discover as much about the person as possible. Obviously in pre-hospital care this is unrealistic; as ambulance clinicians you make guesses or predictions about others, based on your own socialization and your own experiences. Being aware of how we are socialized into society should enable you as ambulance clinicians to appreciate the influences on development of identity and challenge your first impressions of members of society.

Stop and think – What factors influence the first impressions you have when you arrive on scene, when at work?

Having briefly explored how we develop our own identities it is logical to explore our position in society and introduce some sociological concepts/approaches.

Social stratification

Definition of inequality

Inequality refers to differences between people in terms of their abilities and rewards (Marsh and Keating 2006: 206).

Crompton (1989) suggests that inequality leads to social stratification – members of society being ranked in a hierarchical manner. This ranking system depends on factors such as income, wealth, age, power, status and gender. The importance of inequality must not be underestimated; it has been the subject of much research and profoundly affects a person's quality of life and can specifically affect the length of life (Bartley 2004).

Link to Chapter 12, pages 191–3, for more detailed reading about inequality and mortality.

A term that students may be more familiar with is that of social class. Prior to indus-trialization, societies were relatively closed. This refers to people not really moving far from where they were born and not having any other prospects, other than those associated with the social group they were born into. Marsh and Keating (2006) state that with industrialization a more open system developed, due to competition and more opportunity for social mobility. It is commonly accepted by sociologists that modern societies are stratified on the basis of social class (Crompton 1989).

Stop and think – Would you classify yourself as being from the same social class as your ancestors?

With a stratified approach to society, it is important that we can all explore where we are in the hierarchy. Most people have heard of the five-category Registrar General's scale. Since 1998 this has been superseded by a scale adapted by the Office for National Statistics (ONS) (Box 11.1).

Box 11.1 The ONS socio-economic classification analytic classes (1998)

1.   Higher managerial and professional occupations:
1.1 Large employers and higher managerial occupations
1.2 Higher professional occupations

2.   Lower managerial and professional occupations

3.   Intermediate occupations (e.g. clerks, secretaries, computer operators)

4.   Small employers and own account workers

5.   Lower supervisory and technical occupations

6.   Semi-routine occupations (e.g. cooks, bus drivers, hairdressers, shop assistants)

7.   Routine occupations (e.g. waitresses, cleaners, couriers)

8.   Never worked and long-term unemployed

Source: www.statistics.gov.uk/methods_quality/ns_sec/

Classification systems are rarely perfect and Marsh and Keating (2006) highlight some criticisms of this eight-class scale. Marxist writer Coser (1977) believes a scale does not reflect the relationship between each class and therefore negates the importance of division, conflict and dynamics of class struggle. Other criticisms of a class scale are that variations between occupations are not taken into account. Despite being in the same category, for example, a consultant doctor and a junior doctor do very different jobs and have different standards of living. The scale is based on the working population, so how are retired people and housewives represented? Oakley and Oakley (1981) and Crompton (1989) criticize the scale, as the occupation of the male head of household dictates the category. Feminists propose that a more gendered approach to social scales needs to be considered (Sydie 1987; Maynard 1990; Walby 1990). The terms upper, middle and working classes are still commonly used within society, but are they valid sociological concepts in twenty-first-century Britain?

> Link to pages 165–79 in this chapter to explore the links between all of these factors.

There is no argument that social class affects opportunities and lifestyle for all of us. It is a common perception that we are all able to move up the social class 'ladder', if we have the right conditions to do so (education, employment opportunities, for example). This is commonly referred to as social mobility. One would assume that in twenty-first-century Britain, people have the opportunities to change and shape their lives, so the following news article makes interesting reading.

Education 'fails poorer children'

A cross-party commission should be set up to examine the reasons behind the UK's very low social mobility, an education charity says.

The study found that children born in the 1950s had a better chance of escaping poverty than those born in 1970.

The decline in social mobility seen during the 1970s and 1980s has now flattened off, the report concludes, but shows no sign of reversing.

'The UK comes bottom of the table for developed countries for which there is data available', it adds.

Story from BBC News: www.http://bbc.co.uk/go/pr/fr/-/1/hi/uk/6236108.html (Accessed 29 June 2007)

Gender and sexuality

The inclusion of gender as a factor affecting our socialization is widely accepted by sociologists, although this is a relatively new area (since the mid-1980s) of socio-logical investigation. Feminist writers (Walby 1990; Jackson and Scott 1996) have been concerned about the subordination of women as a result of gender. Marsh and Keating (2006) assert that gender is socially constructed and men and women are gendered beings. All areas of our lives are influenced by our gender, again highlighting the connection between all the social factors discussed in this chapter. Sexuality is also socially constructed. The media are very active in providing examples and meanings of femininity and masculinity; this shapes people's gender identities. Magazines are the key media vehicle that promotes conventional and oppressive meanings about gender and sexuality.

Link to pages 177–8 in this chapter to explore the potential power of the media.

There still remains inequality for women in the household and workplace but the situation has improved over time. Meanings about femininity and masculinity are constructed and reinforced in the labour market place; for example, some jobs are predominantly thought of as masculine (builder, steel worker) and some are thought to be more feminine in nature (waitress, nurse). Fifty-eight per cent of managers and senior managers in the NHS are female, maybe reflecting the fact that 50.2 per cent of NHS managers have a clinical background and maybe at one time were nurses themselves (NHS Confederation 2007).

 Stop and think – How do professions that are thought by many members of the general public to be more male-dominated, such as pre-hospital care, 'treat' women?

Marsh and Keating (2006) suggest health is also gendered. The experience of health, although influenced by biology, is also influenced by the social construction of femininity and masculinity. Our gender also affects our health behaviour (a fact that ambulance clinicians should be aware of) in terms of accessing healthcare professionals and services. Men are less likely to access health promotion services than women. Women visit their general practitioners (GPs) more regularly than men, but women live longer. An awareness of the importance of gender within society is crucial to healthcare professionals when trying to provide appropriate quality care. An awareness of the social construction of gender should assist students to question what they may experience and why. It may also help them to question what they see in society and encourage further reading, as this chapter will only provide an introduction to the areas discussed.

Families and family life

Definition of nuclear family

A *nuclear* family is a household unit composed of a man and a woman in a stable marital relationship and their dependent children (Bilton *et al.* 2002: 230).
This is only one of many available definitions.

One of the areas that significantly affects our socialization is the family and family life. Marsh and Keating (2006) explain that all societies have some form of family arrangement. The values, structure and 'norms' of families and family life vary both culturally and across generations. It is therefore more complex to explain what we mean by 'family' than might be first thought or as the definition above might lead us to believe. We all have our own understanding of what 'family' means to us, but when compared to other definitions it soon becomes clear that there is no agreed definition. The diversity of today's contemporary society, resulting from recent changes in family living involving divorce, cohabitation, remarriage, stepfamilies, lone parents, two career households, to name a few, makes the ability to define 'family' more difficult (Cheal 2002). It is not just about structure but about what people do in the family – caring, fulfilling obligations, for example. This also varies across different cultural groups within society. A broad definition is given by Van Every (1999: 178):

> A household is a residential group whose members usually share some basic tasks (like cooking). A family may or may not also be a household, but is usually distinguished by formal ties of 'blood' and marriage. However, 'family' also denotes ties of love and affection, commitment, and obligations whether these are formally recognized or not.

Link to pages 168–9 of this chapter to explore how culture and families are inextricably linked.

Irrespective of the change in family structure, industrialization prior to and during the 1950s played a part in establishing in family patterns. Prior to the 1950s, households in Britain had strong family networks, as families lived close to each other, providing often daily contact for advice and support. After the 1950s there were many developments in housing conurbations and occupational opportunities, which led to increased distances between family members, resulting in a more nuclear family than ever before and less contact between extended family members (Van Every 1999; Cheal 2002). It is, however, thought that developments in communication and transport have enabled this contact to be renewed to some extent over the 1980s and 1990s.

Stop and think – Would some of the calls you attend be prevented had there been an extended family member present to offer advice? At how many calls you attend, specifically to children, is an elder member of the family present? Do you think this demonstrates the importance of 'extended' family?

Functionalist theorists maintain that the family remains a fundamental feature of society. The family is able to adapt and evolve to meet societal needs. Cheal (2002: 8) defines functionalism as a 'theoretical approach which stresses the positive benefits of families. Families are therefore often described as adaptive systems, which respond creatively to the stresses that are caused by unmet needs.' More negative interpretations of the family provided by conflict theorists, such as Marx (cited in Coser 1977), see the family being about power relationships and social control, and restrictions on the individuality of family members. The issues of domestic violence and child abuse are also family issues which are different areas of social life that ambulance clinicians will face. Theories associated with these subjects require extensive reading from specialist researchers in order for students to have an appreciation of the complex nature of these issues.

Link to Chapter 9 for more information about maintaining child safety and the ambulance clinician's role.

Family patterns are constantly changing as the patterns and trends in divorce and marriage demonstrate (see Box 11.2).

Box 11.2 Marital status 1994–2004

	1994	2004
Total – Males, all ages	24,853	25,989
Single	11,410	12,756
Married	11,432	10,863
Widowed	733	726
Divorced	1,278	1,644
	1994	2004
Total – Females, all ages	26,263	27,057
Single	10,116	11,338
Married	11,600	10,935
Widowed	2,922	2,628
Divorced	1,625	2,156

Source: ONS 2007b

The family is a complex social construct which to some extent influences who we are and is interdependent on some other social factors discussed in this chapter.

Culture

As ambulance clinicians are exposed to wide cultural diversity within twenty-first-century Britain, a sociological understanding of culture may improve your understanding of some central issues. Society and culture are so closely linked that one could not exist in any 'meaningful' way without the other. Marsh and Keating (2006) remind us that what is regarded as normal and acceptable behaviour by one society or cultural group may be punished as a crime in another part of the world. Socialization alone in a child's early years is not sufficient for physical, intellectual, emotional and social development. The quality of a child's cultural experience is crucial for her development, as exhibited by cases of physical child abuse and neglect. Sociologists believe cultural deprivation can help explain differences in patterns of criminal behaviour and educational achievement between varying social groups (Hall 1992).

Link to pages 178–9 in this chapter; Chapter 7 and Chapter 9 for much more detail on all these areas.

The work of Mays and Tutt in the 1950s and 1970s respectively demonstrates that there are links between delinquency, cultural deprivation and a 'lack of satisfactory family life'. Social researchers have been exploring the causes of educational failure. The main bulk of this work was undertaken from the 1920s through to the 1960s and into the 1980s. In Britain, the work of Douglas in 1964 indicated that cultural deprivation was part of the reason for educational under-achievement of children from poor backgrounds. Government reports, such as the Plowden Report in 1967 (Central Advisory Council for Education 1967), indicated that parental attitudes towards education and resources in the home were also a significant factor in educational attainment.

This brief diversion into education demonstrates the interrelationship between many areas of our social lives. Each of us will have varying views on the importance of one area over another, but there can be no argument that culture is one of the areas of our lives that has an impact on subsequent education and employment opportunities. Inequality associated with opportunity is also closely linked to all areas of our lives and requires closer examination.

Link to BBC News article on page 165.

Race

Definition of ethnicity

The cultural identity of particular minority groups (Marsh and Keating 2006: 351).

Marsh and Keating (2006) highlight that there have been numerous attempts by theorists to explain 'race', racism and patterns of racial discrimination from the nineteenth century to today. Theories commenced by highlighting the physical differences between groups of people, so called biological theories. During the 1960s and 1970s differences in personality and social behaviour were explained by socio-biological theories concentrating on genetic differences. As this brief history shows, there have been, and continue to be, a number of sociological theories concerning 'race'. The 'race relations' theory attributes divisions in society to the 'favouritism' of certain ethnic groups over others. Later race theories are termed political or state-centred and explore how social and political policy excludes groups in society that do not conform to norms. This can lead to marginalization of certain groups if, for example, certain groups are categorized as likely to commit certain crimes ('Asian looking males with beards linked with mass terrorism'). Other race theories have examined ethnicity when exploring the differences between white and black people's experiences within society (Wellman 1977; Hall 1992; Sampson 1993 and Cohen 1994). An awareness of the above issues may assist the ambulance clinician to avoid contributing to behaviour that further marginalizes certain racial groups within society. The two most important factors in defining a person's identity are history and culture.

> Link to Chapter 4, pages 34–8, to explore the importance of working in an anti-discriminatory manner.

Despite these numerous theories, racial inequality continues in twenty-first-century Britain. Again, many of the social factors are inextricably linked and are interdependent. A person's social and ethnic background influences educational opportunities and subsequent achievement. Research has proven that African-Caribbean children do less well than the general population at school/college, despite an improvement from earlier studies (Drew and Gray 1991). This may impact on their employment prospects (Marsh and Keating 2006). Considering work/employment, discrimination exists in manual and professional occupations to this day; despite the majority of the black population in Britain having been born and educated here, inequalities still exist.

Education and employment have been discussed and undoubtedly have an impact on housing, another area where there are marked inequalities between different ethnic groups, in particular black and white people. The policy of local government housing departments tends to work more favourably if a family conforms to a structure common among the white population: small, one-generation families. The private housing sector of society tends to direct black people towards less prestigious and 'poorer' areas of a region; this all contributes to reinforcing inequalities and discrimination. Being subject to inequality and discrimination has undoubtedly led to 'racial disturbances' in British cities since the mid-1970s, according to Marsh and Keating (2006). Research has cited deprivation of black people living in rundown inner city areas, a poor relationship with the police and political marginalization of black people as causes for the disturbances.

Religion

The classical sociologists (Durkheim 1954; Weber 1963; Marx, cited in Coser 1977) all took the opportunity to study religion and try to explore its sociological meanings and purpose. These theories have been subsequently developed further by more contemporary colleagues. Durkheim (1954) defined religion as a 'unified system of beliefs and practices relative to sacred things', where followers are bonded into a moral community or church. Once established within society, these beliefs become autonomous in their existence. Weber (1963) theorized there being four main categories of religious organization: the church, denomination, sect and cult. Weber believed religion affected other aspects of society, such as economies, ethics and politics. Building on Weber's ideas, functionalist approaches focused on religion's divisive and integrative effects. Bellah (1967) coined the term 'civil religion'; history in Northern Ireland provides an example of division and conflict based upon religious beliefs.

Definition of Neo-Marxism

School of thought based on the further development of Marxist philosophy (Bilton *et al.* 2002: 545).

Traditional Marxism views religion as very powerful and able to reinforce class division and oppression. Neo-Marxist theorists such as O'Toole (1984) have highlighted that the power of religion can be liberating for some people and cite parts of Africa and Eastern Europe as examples.

Glock and Stark (1968) identified five dimensions of religiosity: belief, practice, experience, knowledge and consequence. Sociologists have attempted to examine the social context and consequences of belief systems, but this can be difficult when considering changes over time and cultural differences. Across the world, religion has a resounding power, both politically and culturally. Secularization had been thought to be a growing movement, but this is yet to be seen across the world as belief systems remain popular and powerful, more so in certain areas of the world than others.

Definition of secular

Not concerned with religion (Bilton *et al.* 2002: 547).

Ambulance clinicians must be mindful that religious beliefs have an effect on patients' views, attitudes and behaviour and that religion is an aspect of a person's 'being' that they should consider and respect.

Education

All of us have varying experiences of our childhood and adolescent schooling, some positive and creative, others negative and destructive. Following the interdependent theme, the influence of our families upon our educational experiences should not be underestimated. Marsh and Keating (2006) suggest that sociologists will not focus on intelligence at birth but the ways families influence educational achievement after birth and the social labelling children experience according to their background. It must also be remembered that children also learn from non-formal educational opportunities, for example parents, friends and the television (Hodge and Tripp 1986; Gunter and McAleer 1990; Newburn and Hagell 1995).

Durkheim (1956) took a structural approach to education and believed it to maintain continuity in society. Marx (cited in Coser 1977) saw the role of education as maintaining continuity but also saw it as a potential source of conflict and change with respect to inequality of opportunity. Marsh and Keating (2006) suggest that sociologists focus upon the ways in which families influence educational achievement after birth and the social labelling children experience according to their background, rather than children's intelligence at birth.

 Stop and think back to your school days. Were inequalities obvious? Were you aware of your social status?

The egalitarian approach to sociology is clear when discussing education. Egalitarianism, as Marsh and Keating (2006: 558) describe, is concerned with

> emphasizing the equality of outcomes, where identifiable social groups are not over or under-represented among high or low achievers. This means that the population of a social group represented among university graduates (and also among those without qualifications) should correspond with the proportion of that group in the whole population.

Such egalitarian arguments support the view that children should be compensated for wider social inequalities by the provision of extra resources and help. However, it is realized that social inequalities cannot be solved by education alone. The debate about educational policy is ongoing and issues such as parental choice and equal access are at the heart of the debate. Since the 1980s, girls have on the whole outperformed boys (DfES 1994), partly, Marsh and Keating (2006) suggest, as a result of an anti-sexist, equal opportunities and wholly egalitarian approach to educational policy. Educational achievement is influenced more by social class than by ethnicity or gender. The issue of ethnicity and education requires further research, as much difficulty has been encountered categorizing individuals and questions that seem to be more about social class than ethnicity. Statistical data is also lacking and areas that have been little researched to date, such as children with a disability, need a more focused, researched approach in order to be understood.

Age

Our social world is structured and ordered by age. At times we may not be able to do something because of our age, for example enter a pub alone under the age of 18 years, or it is more acceptable to behave in a certain way because of our age – a child having a tantrum, for example. We can be both enabled and constrained by our age. Age can be classified in three areas: chronological age, biological age and social age. Our chronological or numerical age results in us being able to access certain privileges and may be linked to laws, for example being able to drink alcohol legally in pubs.

Biological age and chronological age are linked. Biological age is linked to physical appearance. One of the reasons why we are so concerned with our biological age and appearance is centred on society's response to biological age. It is about how you look and the way people respond to the way you look. How a person feels in relation to his age group and life experiences is termed social age. Here, a 70-year-old may biologic-ally look older, but may feel socially 'young' and no different to when he was 40 years of age. Society expects people to act and look their age – hence comments like 'mut-ton dressed as lamb', when an individual acts outside the social norm. An extract from the media highlighting one of the London Borough of Southwark's events as part of their week-long Silver Festival for senior citizens describes the use of the Ministry of Sound nightclub from 13.30–16.30 hours for older residents of the borough to 'reminisce, socialize and maybe have the chance to dance' (Freeman 2007: 17).

The Guardian   Sat. March 31st 2007

ID not required Beat goes on and on at the Ministry of Sound

Nightclub opens for Southwark senior citizens as residents flock to council's festival of old age

Hadley Freeman

The queue outside was as long and impatient as ever. The Ministry of Sound, the legendary south London nightclub, is well used to anxious punters braving all weathers to get inside to dance, drink and maybe make eye contact with a beautiful stranger on the dance floor.

Yesterday was no exception. But instead of Jay-Z's white limo outside there was an Age Concern van; in the vestibule, usually filled with twitchy clubbers, canes, Zimmer frames and wheelchairs clattered together.

Yesterday, between the unusual hours of 1:30 and 4:30 (pm, not am), the Ministry hosted the Silver Social, an afternoon for 450 Southwark council residents over 60 years old 'to reminisce, socialise and maybe have a chance to dance'.

And it was a chance the increasingly impatient clubbers were keen to have.

Clutching her carer's arm as she disembarked from the minivan, Feyidiya Davis, 82, was smiling with excitement. 'I love music, and I'm told there will be some singing, too!' she said. She was particularly hoping to be able to dance to her favourite song, Amazing Grace.

Robert Rider, 69, declared himself more of a Frank Sinatra man: 'Me and my wife have come for an afternoon out. Oh yes, we love music,' he said, tucking his hearing aid carefully behind his ear.

As anyone who has ever tried to organise a big night out knows, there are always logistical problems. Janet James from Stone's End day centre smiled stoically as she tried to steward the queue. 'These events can be difficult. As you see, people have mobility problems.'

Finally the doors opened and the excitement was palpable. At first, it looked as though the nightclub hadn't bothered to make itself over too much for its new style of dancers: the lights were blinding, leading to some wheelchairs banging into the backs of ankles, and the bar, dance room and chillout room were all represented.

But small differences slowly came into focus: the usual leaflets advertising future club nights had been pushed aside for pamphlets from Disabled Living. The bar, it transpired, had been dubbed 'the tea room' and the Southwark residents all calmly took their china cups and sat in circles, a chance to refuel before hitting the dancefloor.

Top 10 Residents' choice

1 **Rock Around the Clock** Bill Haley and the Comets
2 **Let's Twist Again** Chubby Checker
3 **In the Mood** Glen Miller
4 **The Last Waltz** Engelbert Humperdinck
5 **New York, New York** Frank Sinatra
6 **The White Cliffs of Dover** Vera Lynn
7 **(I Can't Get No) Satisfaction** Rolling Stones
8 **Is This the Way to Amarillo** Tony Christie
9 **Jealousy** Frankie Laine
10 **Dancing Queen** Abba

The fact that this was newsworthy emphasizes the fact that this kind of initiative is out of the realms of 'normal' for older members of the population. This publicity may encourage other social and fun activities. Age stratification as a sociological concept refers to the 'unequal distribution of social resources, including wealth, power and status, which are accorded to people on the basis of their age' (Marsh and Keating 2006: 359). Childhood, youth, young adulthood, mid-life and old age are key groupings according to Bradley (1996). Old age and childhood are prime examples from British society where we ascribe less status and value to some age groups, compared with others. Just the titles of some organizations indicate this to be true. Why is there a *National* Society for Prevention of Cruelty to Children (NSPCC) and a *Royal* Society for the Protection of Cruelty to Animals (RSPCA)?

In addition to being a biological process, age is also socially constructed and our experiences of age depend on our society. As with gender, ethnicity and class, age is a social variable. There can also be social divisions associated with age; for example, the experience of ageing for a working-class woman will be very different from the experience of an older middle-class man.

Marsh and Keating (2006) explain that prior to 1990 the sociology of childhood was mainly concerned with the child's future worth as an adult. This changed in the 1990s to focus on the children's present-day lives, not their future as adults. Now sociology takes children's views seriously and considers them to be able to shape their own lives, within certain constraints. There is a dichotomy within society about how children are viewed. On one hand they are seen as vulnerable and innocent, in need of protection from the adult world. On the other hand, they are vulnerable and corruptible and in need of control. Children are subject to many age-based institutions which clearly show the different status given to children and adults, where they learn about power and authority, for example playgroups, nurseries, Cubs/Brownies and youth clubs. These experiences and membership of age-related groups enable children to understand the way society is structured through age. Our perceptions of the very young and very old are shaped by our society. The influences on our perceptions are also interrelated factors, social, political and historical context, language, ideologies and media. The policies and politics associated with a particular age group also influence our thinking; this may change over time. For example, the concept of retirement is generally thought to be positive and associated with enjoyment but many older people find retirement frustrating and boring.

 Stop and think about how children and older people are portrayed on the television.

People can be 'stereotyped' within social groups and this can prevent ambulance clinicians from exploring the wide diversity of experiences or knowledge the person may have. Lives, in any age grouping, will vary according to other variables – class, gender, ethnicity, disability. This stereotyping is reflected in the terminology and language used in society today. Older people are sometimes referred to as 'little old ladies', 'the old boy', 'old biddy', as a few examples.

Link – to Chapter 4 pages 34–9 to read about acceptable practice.

 Stop and think – Do you use such stereotypical language? Would you like it to be used about you as you get older?

In relation to the other variables, women are more likely to live in poverty (as their pensions tend to be less than those of men). Women also tend to live longer than men, meaning they are more likely to end up living alone in later life (Vincent 2003). Ambulance clinicians should respond to all individuals in a professional manner, demonstrating dignity and respect. Exploring the social construction of age and ageing may assist clinicians to question their own practice, language and general approach to people.

Work

As explored earlier, we are all members of many social groupings: parent, daughter/ son, employee, and so on. Thus we often take on different roles such as carer or teacher and we also have hobbies/leisure activities that we pursue. When we are asked 'What do you do?' we almost always refer to our paid employment, the role we fulfil in that aspect of our social world and what we think of as 'our work'. Paid labour is associated with work; for example, teaching your child to read is not considered your work as you are not paid to do it. Your child's teacher is paid for that one aspect of the role and much more besides. The work of Marx (McLellan 2000) is important when trying to explain the value of work in our social world. Marx's concept – mode of production – has two components (McLellan 2000). Marx defined the labour process as the 'manner in which purposeful human activity fashions objects and the tools (referred to as means of production) with which this is done'. The social relations of production refers to 'the relationships that form within and around the labour process' (Marsh and Keating 2006: 139). Marx worked on the concept that a worker sells his labour power as a commodity. Braverman (1974) translated this view into the twentieth century and took the view that workers had become 'deskilled' by management, who were attempting to reduce the power of the workforce and regain control of it. Subsequently, this view has been criticized as being over-simplistic and failing to take into account the employees' resistance to having their 'skill' level reduced or altered.

Industrialization has not brought consistent employment to society. It is commonly thought that industrialization would be the inevitable consequence across the world. In many sectors of industry there has been a rise in unemployment, which has challenged this view. Many people have experienced the depressing experience of unemployment, with rates of employment varying across Britain and for different 'groups' of people. Unemployment is a feature for many modern societies.

From Table 11.1, it can be seen that unemployment rates for Black and Pakistani/ Bangladeshi people were three times greater than that for White people, and the rate

Table 11.1 Unemployment rates: by ethnic group and age, 2000–01, United Kingdom in % of ethnic group

	16–24 years	25–34 years	35–44 years	45–59/64 years	All aged 16–59/64
White	11	5	4	4	5
Black	32	14	11	10	15
Indian	13	5	7	6	7
Pakistani/Bangladeshi	28	14	12	–	17
Other groups	24	9	11	7	12
All ethnic groups, including those who did not state ethnic group	12	5	4	4	6

Source: ONS (2003)

for other minority ethnic groups was more than twice that for White people. For all ethnic groups, unemployment is much higher amongst young people aged 16 to 24 than for other age groups. Nearly one-third of young Black people were unemployed, and only a slightly lower proportion of Pakistani/Bangladeshi young people. However, the unemployment rates among Indian people were only slightly higher than those for White people at all ages.

The unemployed can be assigned a social class based on their previous occupation. Unemployment rates for people from minority ethnic groups in the top four social classes were, on average, more than twice those for White people in 1998–2000. The differential was less for the partly skilled, at six percentage points and among the unskilled the difference was four percentage points (ONS 2003). It is not only ethnic origin that has a part to play in unemployment rates; it seems where you live is a factor too. Differences in unemployment rates within regions are greater than differences between regions. In the 12 months ending December 2006, the region with the greatest contrast between local authorities was London, with over 10 percentage points between the areas with highest and lowest unemployment rates. In London the highest unemployment rate is in Tower Hamlets at 14.2 per cent and the lowest rate is in Richmond-upon-Thames at 4.1 per cent (ONS 2007a). As can be seen by a brief overview of the figures, many aspects of unemployment are inextricably linked – a thread of this chapter.

For the majority of the population, who are employed, their rights and protection may be looked after by the trade unions. Although the role of trade unions has changed over time, due to changing socio-economic conditions, they are a crucial part of our society. Millions of workers benefit from the function of trade unions, despite some hostile legislation and efforts by large transnational corporations to reduce the power of the unions. The concept of capitalism is now worldwide, no longer a regional or country-wide phenomenon. Sophisticated technology, satellite and telecommunication systems have enabled production, trade and finance to be organized at a global level. The power of the transnational corporations must not be negated, as we all feel the influence, no matter where we are in the world.

The mass media

Any healthcare professional is subject to the portrayal of his job in the media; ambulance clinicians are no different. How many of you have been called 'Josh' or had your entire career compared to one exciting hour per week in the BBC television show *Casualty*? Television is one aspect of the media that forms part of our everyday lives. The media provide entertainment and information to the large majority of the British population. People have more choice with television than ever before, with the advances in technology and expansion in the number of channels. The potential power of the media has long been recognized by the government and Marsh and Keating (2006) suggest legal controls, regulations and political restrictions have been imposed on the media, in order to control the mass media influence on society.

The relationship between the media and society has been studied by numerous sociologists, who tend to take either an optimistic or more negative view of the media. In an optimistic vein, our ability to access a greater choice of material to hear, read and view, and more information than ever before is seen as positive. Those with more negative views are concerned about the potential danger of the media being used to manipulate and control societal thinking and actions. Further research examining the link between media input and behaviour is inconclusive, for example research into whether children's television viewing makes them behave violently. It is generally agreed that the media has an influence on society in terms of what we see, hear and read, but this may not have an effect on our behaviour, (Hodge and Tripp 1986; Cumberbatch and Howitt 1989; Gunter and McAleer 1990; Newburn and Hagell 1995).

It is clear that in twenty-first-century Britain, society is more informed than ever before. The media play a part in all our lives – how our jobs are perceived, how our profession is perceived, how our organization is perceived. The influence of the media can be on a macro scale, as with nationally broadcast stories, serials, newspapers, or can be more micro, focusing on local stories that hit the local newspaper headlines. This has implications for workers in public services, as very often what is portrayed in the media can affect the public's perception of the service and the care the individual will receive from the NHS Trust or organization concerned.

Crime

In the course of your duties you will come across criminal behaviour by some members of society and you will be involved in circumstances where the police are present. The mere presence of police suggests a visible presence of social control. As members of another uniformed service, it is likely that ambulance clinicians may also be associated by some members of the public with a form of control. It is wise to be aware of this perception, in order to anticipate potential verbal and/or physical abuse; it may help you to take steps to protect yourself and your colleagues. It is recognized by sociologists that a 'police culture' has contributed to segregation of specific sections of society, particularly young black people (Marsh and Keating 2006).

 Stop and think – Have you been subject to verbal and/or physical abuse while at work? Were the police present or not? Do you think the police presence may have made the situation worse?

In the view of most members of society, crime has increased in Britain during the twentieth century. Statistics show that crime is mostly committed by males. Ethnic minorities, specifically black males, are more likely to be convicted and punished for crimes than any other social group (Home Office 2000 and 2003; Home Office/ Office of National Statistics 2007). Sociologists warn not to be overwhelmed by the statistics, pointing out that the police are better equipped and there are many more laws now than earlier in the twentieth century, hence more information is known about crime and more crimes are punished. Also the role of the mass media cannot be negated in raising the public's awareness of criminal behaviour and associated statistics.

Crime is not just observable in adults. Campbell (2007) cites the murder of the toddler James Bulger by two teenagers as being instrumental in the move towards criminalization of children by British society. At this time, Tony Blair coined the phrase, 'tough on crime, tough on the causes of crime' (Campbell 2007: 14) to reassure society that this degradation of moral and social conduct would not be tolerated and would be punished. This stance has not changed, Campbell (2007: 15) writes: 'The last three years has seen a 26 per cent increase in the numbers of children and young people criminalized and seven times as much is spent on youth custody as on prevention schemes. We lock up 23 children per 100,000 population, compared with six in France, two in Spain, 0.2 in Finland.' One reason why so many children are criminalized in the UK, compared to other European countries, may be because the crime seen and experienced by the general public is generalized disturbance and crime in public spaces, which affects people's quality of life and a large number of people. This has changed from individuals being affected by crimes, such as burglary, which do not affect a large number of people at one time. Hence, people are gathering together and applying pressure on their local MPs to increase punishment, which eventually reaches the higher echelons of the government and justice system.

Crime is beyond the realms of other deviant behaviours, as it is punishable by criminal law. People who break the law generally want to keep this area of their lives secret, so it is difficult to research and obtain accurate and reliable data. A number of explanations for people committing crime have been suggested, leading to a range of sociological perspectives being developed. I hope that this brief discussion may encourage you to explore the subject of crime further.

Conclusion

I hope that your awareness of the importance of each of the areas mentioned above has widened your view of your own world and that of others. This chapter has asked clinicians to stop and think about their own personal and working lives, in an attempt to make the theory more relevant to practice. It has introduced you to various sociological theorists and demonstrated the value of understanding how theory can impact practice.

Chapter key points

- The process of socialization occurs at various points in all of our lives.
- Socialization by primary and secondary groups influences our identity.
- Social stratification is explained in terms of socio-economic groups and occupations.
- There are numerous areas of our lives that can be examined from a sociological perspective and you are encouraged to examine your own beliefs, judgements and behaviour.
- Most areas of our lives can be examined in sociological terms. There are areas that we cannot easily change and have 'grown up' with, such as gender, families, age, race, culture, religion and the influence of mass media.

- There are areas of our lives that can be described as transient and are subject to change more readily, such as education, work and crime.

- All of these aspects of our lives are interdependent and inextricably linked.

- Socialization of ourselves and our families may mean that change is much harder to achieve, due to social, economic and political factors.

References and suggested reading

Bartley, M. (2004) *Health Inequality. An Introduction to Theories, Concepts and Methods.* London: Polity Press.

Bellah, R. (1967) Civil religion in America, *Daedalus* 96: 1–21.

Bilton, T., Bonnett, K., Jones, P., Lawson, T., Skinner, D., Stanworth, M. and Webster, A. (2002) *Introductory Sociology*, 4th edn. Basingstoke: Palgrave Macmillan.

Blauner, R. (1972) *Racial Oppression in America.* New York: Harper and Row.

Bradley, H. (1996) *Fractured Identities: Changing Patterns of Inequality.* Polity Cambridge: Press.

Braverman, H. (1974) *Labour and Monopoly Capital: The Degradation of Work within the Twentieth Century.* New York: Monthly Review.

British Broadcasting Corporation (2007) Education 'fails poorer children' BBC News, www.http://bbc.co.uk/go/pr/fr/-/1/hi/uk/6236108.html (Accessed 29 June 2007.)

Brod, H. and Kaufman, M. (1994) (eds) *Theorizing Masculinity.* London: Sage Publications.

Campbell, D. (2007) Bulger, Blunkett, and the making of a 'prison fetish', *Guardian*, 31 March: 14–15.

Central Advisory Council for Education (1967) *Children and their Primary Schools* (Plowden Report). London: HMSO.

Cheal, D. (2002) *Sociology of Family Life.* Basingstoke: Palgrave Macmillan.

Cohen, R. (1994) *Frontiers of Identity: The British and the Others.* London: Longman.

Coser, L.A. (1977) *Masters of Sociological Thought: Ideas in Historical and Social Context.* New York: Harcourt Brace.

Crompton, R. (1989) Class theory and gender, *British Journal of Sociology*, 40 (4): 565–87.

Cumberbatch, F. and Howitt, D. (1989) *A Measure of Uncertainty: The Effects of the Mass Media.* London: John Libbey.

Department for Education and Skills (1994) *Social Trends*, Chart 3.16. London: DfES.

Drew, D. and Gray, J. (1991) The black–white gap in examination results: a statistical critique of a decade's research, *New Community*, 17 (2): 159–72.

Douglas, J.W.B. (1964) *The Home and the School.* London: MacGibbon and Kee.

Durkheim, E. (1954) *The Elementary Forms of Religious Life.* New York: The Free Press.

Durkheim, E. (1956) *Education and Sociology.* New York: The Free Press.

Field, F. (1989) *Losing Out: The Emergence of Britain's Underclass.* Oxford: Blackwell.

Freeman, H. (2007) ID not required. Beat goes on and on at the Ministry of Sound, *Guardian*, 31 March: 17.

Giddens, A. (1973) *The Class Structure of the Advanced Societies.* London: Hutchinson.

Glock, C.Y. and Stark, R. (1968) Dimensions of religious commitment, in R. Robinson (ed.) *Sociology of Religion.* Harmondsworth: Penguin.

Goffman, E. (1963) *Stigma: Notes on the Management of Spoiled Identity.* New York: Prentice-Hall.

Gunter, B. and McAleer, J. (1990) *Children and Television: The One Eyed Monster.* London: Routledge.

Hall, S. (1992) New ethnicities, in J. Donals and A. Rattansi (eds) *Race, Culture and Difference.* London: Sage Publications / Open University Press.

Hall, S., Critcher, C., Jefferson, T., Clarke, J. and Roberts, B. (1978) *Policing the Crisis: Mugging, the State and Law and Order*. London: Macmillan.

Hodge, B. and Tripp, D. (1986) *Children's Television*. Cambridge: Polity Press.

Home Office (2000) *Review of Crime Statistics: A Discussion Document*. London: Home Office.

Home Office (2003) *Home Office Statistics on Race and the Criminal Justice System*. London: Home Office.

Home Office/Office of National Statistics (2007) *Crime in England and Wales 2006/07. A Summary of the Main Figures*, 4th edn. London: Home Office.

Jackson, S. and Scott, S. (eds) (1996) *Feminism and Sexuality: A Reader*. Edinburgh: Edinburgh University Press.

Kornblum, W. (1997) *Sociology in a Changing World*. New York: Harcourt Brace.

McLellan, D. (ed.) (2000) *Karl Marx: Selected Writings*. Oxford: Oxford University Press.

Marsh, I. and Keating, M. (2006) *Sociology: Making Sense of Society*, 3rd edn. London: Pearson Education/Prentice-Hall.

Maynard, M. (1990) The reshaping of sociology? Trends in the study of gender, *Sociology*, 24 (2): 269–90.

Mays, J.B. (1954) *Growing Up in the City*. Liverpool: University of Liverpool Press.

Mead, G.H. ([1934] 1967) *Mind, Self and Society: Works of George Herbert Mead, 1934, from the Standpoint of a Social Behaviourist*. Edited and with an introduction by Charles. W. Morris. Chicago, IL: University of Chicago Press.

Newburn, T. and Hagell, A. (1995) Violence on screen: just child's play, *Sociology Review*, February: 7–10.

NHS Confederation (2007) *Key Statistics on the NHS*. London: NHS Confederation, www//nhsconfed.org/about/about-1857.cfm. (Accessed 9 August 2007.)

Oakley, A. and Oakley, R. (1981) Sexism in official statistics, in J. Irvine, I. Miles and J. Evans (eds) *Demystifying Social Statistics*. London: Pluto Press.

Observer (2000) Road to recovery, *Observer*, 24 September, www.http://observer.guardian-.co.uk/life/story/o,,372311,00.html. (Accessed 2 July 2007.)

Office for National Statistics (2003) *Labour Force Survey*. London: ONS.

Office for National Statistics (2007a) *Labour Market. Local Unemployment Range*. London: ONS.

Office for National Statistics (2007b) *Marriage, Divorce and Adoption Statistics. Review of Registrar General on Marriages and Divorces in 2004, and Adoptions 2005, in England and Wales*. National Statistics Series FM2, No.32. London: TSO.

O'Toole, R. (1984) *Religion: Classic Sociological Approaches*. Ontario: McGraw-Hill.

Ritzer, G. (1996) *Sociological Theory*. New York: McGraw-Hill.

Runciman, W.G. (1990) How many classes are there in contemporary society? *Sociology*, 24: 377–96.

Sampson, E.E. (1993) *Celebrating the Other: A Dialogic Account of Human Nature*. Hemel Hempstead: Harvester Wheatsheaf.

Sivanandan, A. (1982) *A Different Hunger: Writings on Black Resistance*. London: Pluto.

Sydie, R. (1987) *Natural Women, Cultured Men*. Milton Keynes: Open University Press.

The Stationery Office (2007) *Marriage, Divorce and Adoption Statistics. Review of Registrar General on Marriage and Divorces in 2004, and Adoptions 2005, in England and Wales. National Statistics Series FM2. No 32*. London: TSO.

Tutt, N. (1974) *Care or Custody: Community Homes and the Treatment of Delinquency*. London: Dartford Longmann and Todd.

Van Every, J. (1999) From modern nuclear family households to postmodern diversity? The sociological construction of 'families', in G. Jagger and C. Wright (eds) *Changing Family Values*. London: Routledge.

Vincent, J. (2003) *Old Age*. London: Routledge.
Walby, S. (1990) *Theorizing Patriarchy*. Oxford: Blackwell.
Weber, M. (1963) *The Sociology of Religion*. Boston, MA: Beacon.
Wellman, D. (1977) *Portraits of White Racism*. Cambridge: Cambridge University Press.

Useful websites

Age concern: www.ace.org.uk
Department for Education and Skills: www.dfes.gov.uk/childrenandfamilies
Office for National Statistics: www.statistics.gov

12

Psycho-social aspects of health and illness: an introduction
Amanda Blaber

Topics covered:

- Introduction
- Meaning of 'health'
- Sick role
- Stigma
- Chronic illness
- Role of institutions
- Perceptions of illness
- Inequalities
- Conclusion
- Chapter key points
- References and suggested reading

Introduction

Having briefly discussed the main areas that affect our socialization, experience of life and society, it is important to look at our experience of health and illness within twenty-first-century society and to introduce how sociologists and psychologists perceive what is fundamentally the ambulance clinician's area of *business* – ill health.

Meaning of 'health'

Before attempting to explain people's health behaviours it is essential to establish what is meant by 'health'. Blaxter (1990) found that people talked about health in one of three ways. If people saw health as the absence of disease, with no symptoms of illness, Blaxter (1990) termed this a negative definition. Often people describe their health in terms of abilities, for example 'I go to work.' These functional definitions are centred around people being able to carry out their normal activities. Blaxter (1990) considered more positive definitions to be when people concentrated on feeling fit, strong or full of life, in addition to not having any symptoms of illness or a disease. As Denny and Earle (2006) recognize, some sociologists have focused their attention and skills on examining the social factors influencing health and disease; others look at ill health and the patient experience.

From a psychological perspective, Marks *et al.* (2005: 8) define health psychology as 'an interdisciplinary field concerned with the application of psychological knowledge and techniques to health, illness and health care'. This definition is less complicated than the official definition adopted by the American Psychological Association (APA) and the British Psychological Society (BPS), developed by Matarazzo (1982: 4):

> Health psychology is the aggregate of the specific educational, scientific, and professional contributions of the discipline of psychology to the promotion and maintenance of health, the prevention and treatment of illness, the identification of aetiologic and diagnostic correlates of health, illness, and related dysfunction and to the analysis and improvement of the health care system and health policy formation.

The growth of an awareness of both psychological and social influences on health and illness has resulted from the growing disenchantment with the medical model approach (Marks *et al.* 2005). This chapter will explore some key concepts of psychology and sociology that are associated with health and illness; this will introduce the reader to some of the main researchers and writers on the subjects covered. Further reading should be undertaken to develop a better understanding; the suggested reading should be a starting point.

A commonly quoted definition of health is that of the World Health Organisation (WHO) from 1978. It summarizes Blaxter's (1990) findings: 'A state of complete physical, mental and social well-being, and not merely the absence of disease or infirmity.' Other factors such as culture, our experiences and social circumstances can also have a profound effect on our health and our perception of health and illness. Marks *et al.* (2005) believe that there are four approaches to health psychology that are evolving; they represent this visually, as Figure 12.1 shows.

Figure 12.1 shows the four evolving approaches of health psychology, each approach involving research, theory and recommendations for practice. The figure clearly demonstrates the inextricably linked areas of health psychology; each area requires further reading and investigation. Marsh and Keating (2006), taking a more sociological perspective, illustrate that biomedical concepts of health are only one way of looking at health, albeit the most dominant concept in Britain. This is demonstrated by the terminology 'complementary' and 'alternative' medicine to describe other systems/approaches to health care. Within this biomedical approach, patients can have absence of a recognizable disease but have symptoms, such as headache, tiredness or nausea. In terms of modern medicine, Marsh and Keating (2006) suggest that doctors are mechanics to repair a part of our body that has *broken down* due to illness, but also recognize this as an over-simplified explanation. How individuals respond to being *sick* is of interest to

Clinical health psychology	Public health psychology
Core: Age, sex and hereditary factors + Level 1: Individual lifestyle-treatment; secondary and tertiary prevention	Level 3: Living and working conditions – health education, health promotion and primary prevention
Community health psychology	Critical health psychology
Level 2: Social and community influences – Community action and research	Level 4: General socio-economic, cultural and environmental conditions – critique and design of policies and structures

Figure 12.1 Four approaches to health psychology
Source: Marks (2002a, 2002b)

sociologists and psychologists and may help ambulance clinicians understand people's behaviour.

Sick role

Parsons (1951) explored the behaviour of ill people and professional responses to it as a social phenomenon, rather than a biological cause. He assumed two things: that the 'patient–doctor relationship is a social system', based on appropriate behaviour and concerned with norms, and that 'illness is a deviance and is potentially disruptive to social order'. Coming from a functionalist perspective, Parsons (1951) viewed illness as disrupting the functioning of society, but was intrigued to explore the role of health care in maintaining society's well-being. People cannot contribute to society if they are ill – health is needed to fulfil all of our normal social roles, as parents or workers for instance. Having looked at this macro perspective, Parsons (1951) examined how individuals respond to illness.

The term 'sick role' was coined by Parsons (1951) to describe the way individuals and social institutions concerned with medical care (hospitals, general practitioners) socially sanctioned being ill. Parsons (1951) believed that individuals had two rights and two obligations when in the sick role:

- Individuals' rights are: sick people are allowed to give up their normal activities (going to work, school); they cannot be blamed for their incapacity.
- The two obligations are: to get well as quickly as possible, to seek competent care and cooperate with medical help. Parsons (1951) makes a clear distinction between illness and other types of deviance (crime), as the person is not held responsible.

Marsh and Keating (2006) balance the discussion by noting limitations to Parsons's theory. Long-term health problems, for example diabetes or arthritis, do not *fit* Parsons's ideology, as these illnesses have no cure and the individual cannot be obligated to *get well*. The concept of power is also important when discussing the sick role, as doctors act in a social sense to sanction the sick role and also have legal obligations concerning long-term sick leave or controlling access to financial benefits, on behalf of the government. It seems that many individuals crave legitimization of their illness; doctors and ambulance clinicians may be involved in the process.

Parsons (1951) viewed illness as deviance. This has been criticized as being too simple in its explanation of what can be a complex process in terms of accessing assistance, coming to terms with diagnosis and complying with treatment. If your views are similar to Parsons (1951) then some illnesses will be classified as more 'deviant' than others. The work of Goffman (1963) identified 'stigma' as being a social concept. This is interesting to discuss, while remembering Parsons's (1951) concept of classifying illness as a 'deviance'.

Stigma

Definition of stigma

Unfavourable reactions towards people when they are perceived to possess attributes that are denigrated (Marks *et al.* 2005: 62).

Goffman (1963) identified two kinds of stigma:

- Discrediting or visually obvious stigmas, such as loss of a limb or use of a wheelchair. Stigmas challenge our expectations of 'normal' social interaction and the stigmatized person is unsure of how she will be treated and how she will manage the interaction with the 'normal' person.
- Discreditable stigmas. The stigma is not visually obvious, but may become disruptive if discovered, for example history of mental health problems, epilepsy or having a criminal record.

People who are considered to have a stigma very often find it becomes dominant in their life and social role, so no matter what their other responsibilities (partner, parent, employee) they become defined by their stigmatized role, such as 'a wheelchair user', 'an epileptic'. The use of derogatory language by healthcare professionals sometimes reinforces a person's stigma – 'the stroke patient', 'the alcoholic', for example. Marsh and Keating (2006) also note that attributes that result in stigma in some situations may not be the same in other situations; for example, being a single mother in some cultures or subcultures may be discreditable but is the norm in others, so may not result in stigma. It is also important to acknowledge that people with obvious stigmas may pose difficulty for the ambulance clinician, especially if they have little experience of dealing with the general public and are new to health care. It is vital that interpersonal communication skills are practised and that difficult situations are reflected upon, in order that clinicians can improve their interpersonal skills and approach to members of the public in a non-judgemental, confident and professional manner.

Links to Chapter 3, Chapter 4, pages 34–7 and Chapter 5.

Chronic illness

Chronic illness is a feature of twenty-first-century Britain, as people are living longer. By 2010 the number of people over the age of 65 is predicted to be 483,000. By 2020 it is expected to reach 2,351,000 (NHS Confederation 2007). Many people experience the symptoms of chronic conditions; these vary widely but Marsh and Keating (2006: 399) suggest that chronic diseases do share certain features:

- they present long-term health problems;
- they often present multiple health problems;
- there is usually no 'cure', only treatment for symptoms;
- there may be uncertainty about how illness will progress and when;
- they potentially cause major disruption to the lives of sufferers and their families.

Charmaz (1983) describes a *loss of self* as being a central feature of people who experience chronic conditions. An individual's confidence and self-worth are affected. The stigma associated with their chronic condition may mean they distance themselves from social interaction, leading to a negative vicious circle. In describing the sick role, Parsons (1951) considered the individual to be passive and seeking medical help, but many individuals with chronic illness will be 'experts' concerning their condition and a valuable source of information and learning for the ambulance clinician. It is crucial that the ambulance clinician respects and values the individual's expertise and uses the patient's knowledge to learn from him and provide quality care for him. It must also be remembered that people living with chronic illness often have to 'juggle' relationships with health professionals, family and friends, requiring many adaptations and adjustments. Marks *et al.* (2005) describe how psycho-social interventions can help: these range from counselling, psychotherapy or cognitive behaviour therapy to group support or relaxation techniques.

When discussing disability, disability activists (Swain *et al.* 1993; Oliver 1996) advocate the move away from a medical model where the focus is to cure or care and return the individual to *normal*. The focus should be on moving towards a social model, where restrictions within society that disable the individual, for example lack of access to buildings and public transport, are addressed. The social model encourages society to reduce oppression for people with a disability, enabling them to participate in society and reduce oppression via appropriate social policies (Oliver 1996).

Role of institutions

In Britain, while there is much care occurring in the community and in home environments, much health and social care occurs in some type of institution, for example hospices, hospitals, general practitioner surgeries. Foucault (1976) believed hospitals were one type of institution where the state could control the population. Another of Goffman's (1968) studies was asylums, in which he studied the behaviour of staff and inmates in a variety of institutions. The work makes disturbing reading and comments strongly on the power relations in any institution where a group of professionals have power and control over another group of people – patients, for example. Goffman's work is seminal and links well to the discussion of power later in this chapter. Other institutions are the school and prison. However, with the recent reduction in number of hospital beds and reduced length of hospital stay, this challenges Foucault's view, as the focus for twenty-first-century Britain is on the development of primary care. Kleinmann (1978) developed a model of healthcare systems that is applicable to health care in Britain; see Figure 12.2. It is clear from Kleinmann's (1978) model that the sectors of health care identified are distinct and perform different roles within the healthcare system. However, the three areas also overlap; the ideal focus should be on providing the most appropriate care for the patient and not on boundaries. Many individuals are in a position to make informed decisions for themselves – improved access to information through the internet is a significant factor here. It must also be remembered that technology has the potential to widen the inequality gap, for example if people do not have access to a computer or the internet. Healthcare professionals should not assume all their patients have computer access. It must be remembered that not all patients have equality concerning their healthcare decision making, either due to educational opportunities, access to healthcare or financial constraints.

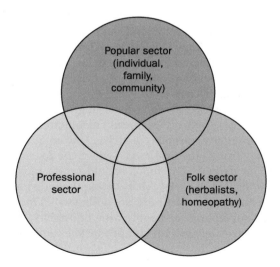

Figure 12.2 Kleinmann's model of healthcare sectors (1978)

Sociologists have considered how and when people make the decision to seek professional help. The work of Kasl and Cobb (1966) reviewed the literature, finding that the severity of symptoms plays only a small part in people's decision making. There are many other factors that an individual considers before seeking help, as shown in Kasl and Cobb's model of illness behaviour (1966).

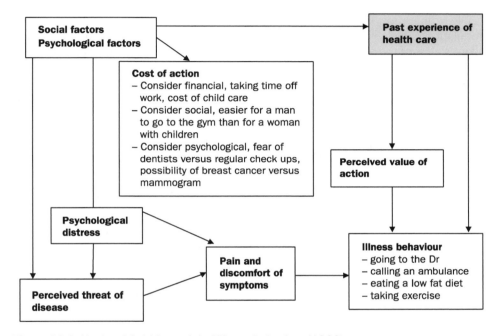

Figure 12.3 Kasl and Cobb's model of illness behaviour (1966)

A person's past experience of health care is highlighted in the tinted box on the diagram, as this is an area where healthcare professionals have the opportunity to make a difference. The work of Goffman (1971) explained how we use props in our daily work, ranging from clothes and stethoscopes to sunglasses and hairstyle to portray the public image we each wish to create and present. Each profession has its own set of props and behaviour into which newcomers are initiated and socialized, not through a formal process or formal instruction but through a process called 'modelling'.

 Stop and think – When you joined the ambulance service, how did you become socialized? Is your public image the same as that of other colleagues?

One reason for mentioning this in this paragraph is that if we know and understand how these processes occur and recognize these aspects in our own behaviour, we can seek to modify our behaviour and image, as appropriate. If you recognize a behaviour that might have affected a person's past experience of ambulance clinicians, you are in a position to alter your public image and improve the client's view and experience of the pre-hospital care service.

Perceptions of illness

Sociological and psychological factors have been discussed in the relevant chapters. Ambulance clinicians and other healthcare professionals can profoundly affect a patient's view of the healthcare system and can influence their decision making about whether to access/seek assistance. It must not be underestimated how much power healthcare professions are able to exert, either implicitly or explicitly.

Balient (1964), using a psychoanalytic approach, researched the doctor–patient interaction and examined communication between the two parties, highlighting the power relations between the two groups. This early research assumed that, in a meeting, the doctor was tasked to uncover the real problem, from the patient's presentation. Balient (1964) believed that the patient attempted to mask the real problem, in a way to test the doctor's expertise. A later study, by, Byrne and Long (1976), identified doctors' varying communication styles. They identified four diagnostic styles and seven prescriptive styles used by the doctors. Briefly, these styles constitute a continuum from patient-centred to doctor-centred styles. The more doctor-centred the interaction, the more power was asserted. Consequently, Kreps (1996) advocated a consumer orientation to health care, in order to address the imbalance of power between providers and consumers. The lack of research concerning other healthcare professionals and power may be an area for further research. Ambulance clinicians must always be mindful of the potential to abuse their power. This is both unprofessional and contradicts the paramedic standards of proficiency (HPC 2007). It is equally important to act as the patient's advocate if you believe a colleague to be abusing the power relationship she has with a patient. The following clarification of the characteristics possessed by a profession makes this discussion clearer.

 Stop and think – Have you witnessed a colleague abuse his position of power? How might this experience affect a person's decision making to access health care in the future? What should you do if you witness a colleague abusing her position of power, or are involved in some way?

Link to Chapter 3.

The superiority of the medical profession within the sphere of health care has been explored by sociologists and psychologists. They concur that a professional has distinct characteristics:

- a specialized body of knowledge;

- a monopoly of practice;
- autonomy to define the boundaries and the nature of her work;
- a code of ethics which regulates relationships both between professionals and between professionals and their clients.

(Marsh and Keating 2006: 412)

Although this distinctly refers to the medical profession, some of these characteristics are common to any healthcare profession. The paramedic profession is no exception.

Definition of iatrogenic illness

Illness or disability caused by medical treatment (Bilton 2002: 543).

Illich (1975) argued that medicine had the potential to make us ill, via side effects and post-operative complications. Illich (1975) called this process iatrogenesis and believed medicine to be too dominant in social and moral life, characterized by medicalization of our lives – for example, drunkenness becomes alcoholism. Illich (1975) would argue that the prevalence of methicillin resistant staphylococcus aureus (MRSA) in many of Britain's hospitals is a result of the medicalization of our lives, as doctors have prescribed antibiotics inappropriately in some cases, leading to the origins of MRSA as an antibiotic-resistant bacterium. Illich (1975) would suggest that MRSA is a direct result of the dominant nature of the medical profession within society.

Inequalities

There are still many areas of life where inequalities exist and affect the health of the population. Inequalities in health and premature death have become a feature of sociologists' and psychologists' work prior to, and after, the Black Report (Townsend et al. 1988), which suggested that inequalities were real and in some areas widening. Successive governments have attempted to develop social policy to try and reduce inequalities, but as inequalities are inextricably linked with other areas of social life this is proving exceedingly difficult. Ethnicity adversely affects health. Sociologists and psychologists have explored the prerequisites of good health (access to jobs, education and quality housing) and their impact on health. Racism affects the access to, and quality of, service received. Gender, as a social construction, affects what we expect of men and women in terms of health (Ogden 2000; Payne and Walker 2000; Bartley 2004). The Office for National Statistics (2004) states that people have been living longer since the 1980s, but not all of these years are in good health, as Figure 12.4 shows.

Women can expect to live longer, but in poorer health than men, as seen in Figure 12.4. Life expectancy is higher for females than for males. In 2001 the life expectancy at birth of females was 80.4 years compared with 75.7 years for males.

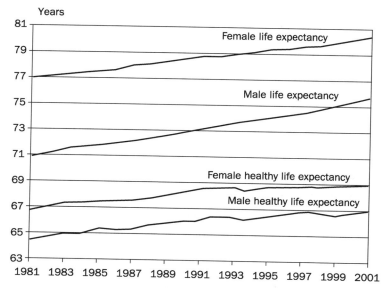

Figure 12.4 Life expectancy and healthy life expectancy at age 65: by sex
Source: Office for National Statistics (2004)

Life expectancy for males has been increasing faster than for females. There was an increase of 4.8 years in male life expectancy between 1981 and 2001. For females the corresponding increase was 3.6 years. Healthy life expectancy for men at age 65 has also increased faster than for women. In the 20 years to 2001 the expected number of further healthy years of life for men aged 65 rose by 1.7 years to 11.6 years. For women there was a rise of 1.3 years to 13.2 years (ONS 2004). It is not only age where inequality can be discussed. The nature of the work we do can also have an impact on our health, as the following edited press extract by Prentis (2005) clearly illustrates:

Cloud cuckoo land

Making NHS staff work longer for their pensions will endanger patients and end up costing the health service more, says Dave Prentis.

The government seems hellbent on alienating public sector workers by attacking hard-won pension rights. Hot on the heels of attacks on the local government pension scheme – to be introduced on April 1 this year – health workers are next in the firing line and are to be forced to work longer for less pension.

People don't go to work in the NHS for the perks or bonuses because there aren't any. But one thing they were always able to rely on was an adequate pension at the end of their working lives. The NHS pension scheme was tried and trusted. It didn't provide a king's ransom, but it provided security and a buffer against poverty in old age where workers may become dependent on means-tested benefits.

To suggest that NHS workers should be forced to work until they are 65 is living in cloud cuckoo land. As it is 73 per cent of paramedics are forced to retire through ill-health before they reach the age of 60, let alone carry on until they are 65. Forcing staff to work longer will simply raise the level of ill-health retirements and end up costing the NHS more.

And what about the possible risk to patients? People whose capability is compromised by age-related problems, but are not eligible for ill-health retirement, may continue to work in vital occupations in order to avoid reducing their pension benefits. This cannot be right and will undermine patient care.

It must be recognized that working for the NHS is physically, mentally and emotionally demanding. It is a highly stressful environment because of the rapid changes in technology; the rapid turnover of patients and constant reforms and changes.

It is essential to take a long view when looking at pensions, but these changes are being driven by short-term cost cutting and not what is in the best interests of health workers, patients and the future NHS.

Dave Prentis is general secretary of public sector union Unison.

(Prentis 2005)

This press extract discusses a very specific inequality. Inequalities in health and illness exist; they are not only related to social class, but exist in all areas of life. Indeed, all areas of our lives are inextricably linked, in health and in our experience of and predisposition to illness. This serves as a brief introduction to the concept of inequality; please refer to the suggested reading for dedicated books on each of the subjects.

Conclusion

There is no doubt that the discussion of health and illness is complex and subject to many sociological and psychological views/perspectives. This chapter has introduced some of the issues, but it is no substitute for further reading and investigation. I envisage that students will gain an understanding of psychology and sociology and sociological/psychological principles from this discussion and I hope it will act as a catalyst for future enquiry.

Chapter key points

- People have varying views on what constitutes *health*.
- People react in a variety of ways to acute illness and chronic ill health.
- The role of institutions and people's behaviour within 'health' institutions is considered.
- All of the above are considered in terms of sociology and psychological theories and theorists.

References and suggested reading

Balient, M. (1964) *The Doctor, his Patient and the Illness*. New York: International Universities Press.

Bartley, M. (2004) *Health Inequality: An Introduction to Theories, Concepts and Methods*. Cambridge: Polity Press.

Bilton, T., Bonnett, K., Jones, P., Lawson, T., Skinner, D., Stanworth, M. and Webster, A. (2002) *Introductory Sociology*, 4th edn. Basingstoke: Palgrave Macmillan.

Blaxter, M. (1990) *Health and Lifestyles*. London: Routledge.

Byrne, P.S. and Long, B.E.L. (1976) *Doctors Talking to Patients*. London: HMSO.

Charmaz, K. (1983) Loss of self: a fundamental form of suffering in the chronically ill, *Sociology of Health and Illness*, 5(2): 168–95.

Denny, E. and Earle, S. (2006) *Sociology for Nurses*. Cambridge: Polity Press.

Foucault, M. (1976) *The Birth of the Clinic*. London: Tavistock.

Goffman, E. (1963) *Stigma: Notes on the Management of Spoiled Identity*. New York: Prentice-Hall.

Goffman, E. (1968) *Asylums – Essays on the Social Situation of Mental Patients and Other Inmates*. Harmondsworth: Penguin.

Goffman, E. (1971) *The Presentation of Self in Everyday Life*. Harmondsworth: Penguin.

HPC (2007) *Standards of Proficiency: Paramedics*. London: HPC.

Illich, I. (1975) *Medical Nemesis*. London: Calder and Boyars.

Kasl, S.V. and Cobb, S. (1966) Health behaviour, illness behaviour and sick role behaviour, *Archives of Environmental Health*, 12: 246–66.

Kleinmann, A. (1978) Concepts and a model for the comparison of medical systems, *Social Science and Medicine*, 12 (2B): 85–93.

Kreps, G.L. (1996) Promoting a consumer orientation to health care and health promotion, *Journal of Health Psychology*, 1: 41–8.

Marks, D.F. (2002a) *The Health Psychology Reader*. London: Sage Publications.

Marks, D.F. (2002b) Freedom, responsibility and power: contrasting approaches to health psychology, *Journal of Health Psychology*, 7: 5–14.

Marks, D.F., Murray, M., Evans, B., Willig, C., Woodall, C. and Sykes, C.M. (2005) *Health Psychology: Theory, Research and Practice*, 2nd edn. London: Sage Publications.

Marsh, I. and Keating, M. (2006) *Sociology: Making Sense of Society*, 3rd edn. London: Pearson Education/Prentice-Hall.

Matarazzo, J.D. (1982) Behavioral health's challenge to academic, scientific and professional psychology, *American Psychologist*, 37: 1–14.

NHS Confederation (2007) *Key Statistics on the NHS*. London: NHS Confederation.

Ogden, J. (2000) *Health Psychology. A Textbook*, 2nd edn. Buckingham: Open University Press.

Oliver, M. (1996) *Understanding Disability*. London: Macmillan.

Office for National Statistics (2004) *Life Expectancy. Life Expectancy Continues to Rise*. www.statistics.gov.uk/cci/nugget.asp?id=168

Parsons, T. (1951) *The Social System*. London: Routledge and Kegan Paul.

Payne, S. and Walker, J. (2000) *Psychology for Nurses and the Caring Professions*. Buckingham: Open University Press.

Prentis, D. (2005) *Cloud cuckoo land*, Guardian, 12 January. www.guardian.co.uk/print/0,,5101628–103690,00.html. (Accessed 3 July 2007.)

Swain, J., Finkelstein, V., French, S. and Oliver, M. (1993) *Disabling Barriers – Enabling Environments*. London: Sage Publications and Open University Press.

Townsend, P., Davidson, N. and Whitehead, P. (1988) *Inequalities in Health (Black Report)*. Harmondsworth: Pelican.

WHO (World Health Organisation) (1978) *Report of the International Conference on Primary Health Care, Alma Ata*. Geneva: WHO.

13

Social policy relevant to paramedic practice
Amanda Blaber

Topics covered:

- Introduction
- Why is this relevant?
- Importance of policy to practice
- Structure of the Department of Health and other main bodies
- Brief overview of *Our Health, Our Care, Our Say*
- Relevance to ambulance services of *Direction of Travel for Urgent Care: A Discussion Document*
- Relevance to ambulance services of *Emergency Access*
- Conclusion
- Chapter key points
- References and suggested reading

Introduction

The everyday practice of any healthcare professional is guided by social policy. An awareness of social policy is fundamental to ensuring contemporary practitioners who are up to date with policy developments and move with the times in their specific profession.

Why is this relevant?

Policy is being developed and proposed on an almost continual basis by the various bodies associated with pre-hospital care, including the Department of Health and British Paramedic Association (BPA). While some organizations are concerned with policy associated with practice, such as the Joint Royal Colleges Ambulance Liaison Committee (JRCALC) and BPA, others are proposing and shaping pre-hospital care for the future – the Department of Health (DoH). Very often the DoH has representatives of professional bodies on the working parties to ensure representation and collaboration when developing policy documents.

Importance of policy to practice

Clinicians have a choice:

- to let policy be published and subsequent changes be implemented by their Trust without their consultation;

or

- to be aware of proposals being made about future services, ensure they have a chance to comment as professional clinicians and individually secure their future as clinicians ahead of the game and aware of how policy shapes practice.

Clinicians who work in this manner are often able to foresee changes before they happen; this in itself will put them in a much stronger position professionally. Peckham and Meerabeau (2007: 268) support the view that 'Health and social care practitioners need an understanding of why particular services exist, the way they work and what impact they have on the users and people who come into contact with them.' This chapter will also provide a brief summary of the structure of the Department of Health and local structures, as well as an overview of the key policy documents relevant to pre-hospital care professionals at this time. The rate of policy production will mean that clinicians will be required to update themselves on a regular basis.

> Link to Chapter 16 to read about professionals' responsibilities concerning keeping their knowledge current and their own professional development.

Structure of the Department of Health and other main bodies

Before exploring specific social policy in relation to pre-hospital care it is worth explaining the structure of the Department of Health and how establishing policy occurs.

Despite the distinct directorates and divisions, detailed in Figure 13.1, the Department of Health maintains a strong professional contribution to policy making. Numerous civil servants employed by the Department of Health originate from professional backgrounds (Ham 2004). Ham (2004: 143) indicates that on many issues there is a 'partnership between the medical profession and the Department of Health' and that consumer/service user groups have less influence. *Our Health, Our Care, Our Say* (DH 2006a) is maybe an attempt to redress the balance, as this policy document is focused upon views and suggestions from NHS service users. There are other bodies and processes that may influence health policy such as, working groups, inquiries into adverse incidents, advice groups such as the NHS Confederation or the National Institute for Clinical Excellence (NICE). All of these have their part to play

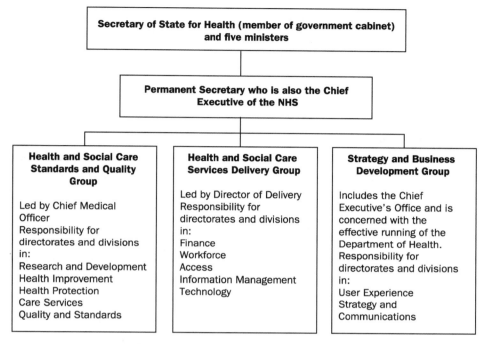

Figure 13.1 Structure of Department of Health and overall responsibilities.
Source: Adapted from Ham (2004: 137)

in defining the NHS of the twenty-first century and the service that it offers to the UK population.

As Ham (2004) states, the Secretary of State relies upon the board of the Strategic Health Authority (SHA) to oversee the commissioning and provision of services locally via the NHS Trusts, Primary Care Trusts (PCTs) and Care Trusts. The SHA is charged with three tasks:

* to create a coherent strategic framework;
* to agree annual performance agreements and performance management;
* to build capacity and support performance improvement.

NHS Trusts are given responsibility for the management of certain services. This varies from Trust to Trust: some run acute hospitals, others manage learning disability, mental health services or ambulance services and others have dual responsibility. PCTs were formed in 2002 and have replaced the Health Authority's function and that of some NHS Trusts. PCTs are responsible for the commissioning of services and managing community services in some parts of the country. Ham (2004) states that with general practitioners (GPs) commissioning services and building upon previous GP fundholding, these clinicians are more directly involved in the management of services than ever before. The implementation of national policies, specifically ones concerned with quality of care, are tasked to PCTs.

Stop and think – In the area in which you live, who is responsible for service provision? Has there been a change in responsibility in recent months? Is the PCT more prevalent than in recent years? Are changes being made to your local acute hospital services?

Definition of Green Paper

Proposals for development of service provision appear first as consultative documents or Green Papers (Ham 2004).

Definition of White Paper

Set out the government's plans for future policy and may be a precursor to legislation (Ham 2004).

From the overview above it is clear that there are numerous bodies involved in the management and regulation of health services, as suggested by Ham (2004). The Department of Health issues guidance on priorities for service development and circulars on a range of topics, explaining national policy which NHS bodies are expected to follow. Some of the circulars are prescriptive and others are advisory in nature. The Department of Health publishes Green Papers, which enable NHS bodies and other interested parties to influence the final definitive White Paper. Doctors are represented at all levels within the Department of Health, the Chief Medical Officer (CMO) being the highest ranking doctor (Ham 2004). Under this Labour government, a number of NHS doctors have been appointed as National Clinical Directors, to lead the Department of Health in priority areas. An example of the appointment of a National Clinical Director is Sir George Alberti, whose proposals will be discussed later in the chapter.

Stop and think – What do you know about recent policy documents? Can you name some? What implications do they have for your daily work?

Brief overview of *Our Health, Our Care, Our Say*

One of the most recent public consultation documents, Our Health, Our Care, Our Say (DoH 2006a), was published after extensive work with service users and represents areas of concern for the general public, community care, hospital care and GP services. It is made very clear that the development of an urgent care strategy for the NHS will 'take full account of the implications for other providers, including social care and ambulance service' (DoH 2006a: paragraph 4.51). This key policy White Paper has led to several subsequent documents that take the areas highlighted and set out proposals for future service development. Examples of these documents are: *Our*

Health, Our Care, Our Say: A New Direction for Community Services (DoH 2006b) and *Our Health, Our Care, Our Say: Making It Happen* (2006c), which provides an update on progress to date. As a result of these documents, new services are being implemented closer to, or in, people's homes, including specific care provided by ambulance clinicians, urgent care centres and rapid response teams, in addition to other health professionals' input. In an attempt to gauge success to date, the National Audit Office (NAO) examined the success of the out of hours services and found that national standards are not being met across England (NAO 2006). *Direction of Travel for Urgent Care: A Discussion Document* (DoH 2006d) has undoubtedly resulted from the NAO report and the findings of *Our Health, Our Care, Our Say* (DoH 2006b), which established that people are not clear about community services in their area or how to access them. The document also aims to explore the fact that urgent or emergency care services are used more by people in deprived areas, 'where primary care services do not adequately reflect need' (DoH 2006d: 1).

Relevance to ambulance services of *Direction of Travel for Urgent Care: A Discussion Document*

The *Direction of Travel for Urgent Care* discussion document (DoH 2006d) discusses three areas: What do service users and carers want? Twenty-first century urgent care, and Turning the model into reality, and includes a fourth section explaining to readers how to comment. Ambulance NHS Trusts are specifically mentioned in relation to providing high-quality cost-effective services. The policy alludes to the development of more community-based services where a 'faster and more convenient' service can be provided. The document recognizes the changing role of ambulance services and the development of emergency care practitioners (ECPs) and differently trained paramedics, enabling the assessment of the patient over the telephone or face to face. The further development of these services may mean there is no need to go to Accident and Emergency (A&E) or be admitted to hospital. In addition to more accurate assessment and autonomy for the clinician, the patient, if hospital treatment is indicated, will be taken not to the nearest facility but to the most appropriate facility with specialist services for her specific requirements. The discussion around these proposals obviously has implications for existing hospitals and, more specifically, A&E departments.

Relevance to ambulance services of *Emergency Access*

If these changes are being driven by 'bringing services to people rather than people to services' (DoH 2006d: 5), a change to the infrastructure of A&E services is required, hence the publication of *Emergency Access* (DoH 2006e), in which Alberti advocates a proposal to 'centralize expertise to provide safer, quicker, more appropriate care for all' (DoH 2006e: 3). At the moment this does not seem to be particularly popular with the public, who wish to protect and keep open their local A&E departments. The DH (2006d: 4) identifies that 'very few people who attend A&E have life-threatening conditions'. It is clear that people require more supportive, accessible primary care 24 hours a day, seven days a week, 365 days a year. Maybe if access to services had been equal across the country, prior to these changes being proposed, the public would be less negative and see the logic of the proposals. The proposals also have implications for resourcing and training for ambulance Trusts and employed clinicians. If frontline vehicles are required to transport patients to specialist/most appropriate facilities, this may involve extended transport times and more intensive treatment en route to the specialist facility. The shape of ambulance services is rapidly changing, with the development of more rapid response units and training of ECPs and paramedic practitioners to fulfil the new roles and to be instrumental in making the new Department of Health-proposed services work. However, the local translation of national Department of Health proposals requires understanding and support from local people.

The strength of feeling about local acute services may have been underestimated. The following news article is a direct result of the proposals made in the *Direction of Travel for Urgent Care* (DH 2006d) document and reflects how these plans have been translated into the West Sussex provision of A&E services. West Sussex PCT have proposed their own local consultation document, *Fit for the Future*, in order to explain their proposals. This is only one example, from one part of England.

Hospital protest heads to London

Campaigners fighting to save their West Sussex hospital from closure are spending the next few days walking to London in protest.

It follows the announcement that two out of the three accident and emergency departments will close in the county.

Supporters of St Richard's Hospital, Chichester, set off on their 76-mile trek to the capital on Thursday.

A&E care at the Worthing and Southlands Hospital, and the Princess Royal, in Haywards Heath, are also in doubt.

West Sussex Primary Care Trust (PCT) announced plans to downgrade two out of the three hospitals on Wednesday.

Westminster petition

Three options, under its *Fit for the Future* consultation, are being considered.

One of the proposals sees St Richard's Hospital losing its A&E department, maternity and complex surgery.

More than 136,000 people have signed a petition to save the hospital.

The petition will be delivered to Downing Street and the Department of Health at the end of the march to London next Tuesday.

It is the second time the protesters have taken their campaign to Westminster.

(BBC 2007)

Stop and think – Have you been asked by patients about your local A&E departments closing? Have you been able to provide accurate and informed information to your patients about changes in service provision?

The alarmingly rapid development and proposals for change within the health service have unfolded while I have been writing this chapter; I have had to review the DoH website weekly in order to check that the chapter is still up to date and relevant. The following article from 17 July 2007 is a clear example of the speed of change. As the comprehensive review and plans for the whole of England by Professor Sir Ara Darzi, Health Minister is not due until the end of 2007, I have decided to include excerpts from a newspaper article relating to the planned changes for London. Please read it and ask yourself questions, in terms of what it will mean for ambulance service provision and for yourselves as ambulance clinicians.

Why Labour's new 'super surgeries' will put lives at risk

David Nunn, consultant orthopaedic surgeon at Guy's and St Thomas's Hospital, London, has 30 years' experience in the capital's hospitals. Here, he warns that new proposals to shut down hospitals in favour of 'super surgeries' have harmed patients before – and will do so again.

In what sounds like the most radical shake-up of the health service for decades, Sir Ara wants to tear up the way the capital is serviced for health care and start again, reducing the number of big hospitals and building a huge network of so-called polyclinics, or super surgeries, instead.

These would handle routine in-patient care, minor A&E services, simple emergency surgery, obstetrics and neonatal care and paediatrics.

They would be staffed by GPs. Meanwhile, consultants would travel between clinics and a reduced number of hospitals, which would simply be open for major elective work or emergency work. The idea is to take the treatment to the patient rather than the other way around, potentially saving money and making medicine more convenient.

As Sir Ara is due to report on his plans for the whole country before the end of the year, you can be sure everyone outside London will be getting something just as dramatic – and horribly similar.

Forgive me if I don't sound thrilled at the thought. It's just that I can recall the same scheme operating 17 years ago – before Labour came to power – and we had to abandon it within a couple of years because it was unwieldy and sometimes dangerous.

Then, super surgeries were staffed by GPs and consultants attended them periodically when needed. But at least we had 'junior staff', who were sufficiently trained to deal with most emergencies if consultants were unable to get to the surgeries.

But with European law restricting the number of hours junior doctors can work, leading to a huge disruption to their training, we no longer have that safeguard.

The most acute problem of creating a whole new class of super surgery or polyclinic – whatever you call them – is the overall effect on Accident and Emergency cover, which will be concentrated in a handful of major A&Es, a pattern that will be repeated across the country.

These departments are already fighting for their existence from Sussex to Yorkshire, and you have to ask whether a reduced number – both in quantity and in size – could handle the consequences of a terrorist attack, rail crash or natural disaster. I doubt we could in London.

When the Soho bomb went off in April 1999, maiming dozens and killing three, we were proud that we could assemble five surgical teams covering all specialities at St Thomas's in one hour from the call coming into A&E. By 8pm that Friday evening, we had nearly 20 consultants ready to operate.

Similarly with the 7/7 bombings, the hospital's major incident plan was put into effect in minutes.

That couldn't have happened under the new plans – we'd all be too far away from our base hospitals to get back and be useful.

When Alan Johnson, our new Secretary of State for Health, made a speech two weeks ago promising to slow down the process of change, on the grounds that NHS staff had been put through enough, I don't think many of us really believed him.

But to see his right-hand man – an academic specializing in robotic keyhole surgery – less than a week later drive a coach and horses through everything we have done and learned in the past twenty years really is too much.

It will be cumbersome, dangerous and expensive. And who will pay for it? I'm afraid once again, it will be the patients.

(Nunn 2007)

This article contains some personal views that are obviously related to many years of experience and reform. Let us take a moment to consider the possible consequences of these proposed reforms for London in terms of ambulance provision and cover:

- Would ambulances be permitted to call at these polyclinics or super surgeries, or would you have to convey patients to the major A&E departments?

- What would this mean for travelling times?

- Would you or the service have to defend your decision about what facility the patient was taken to?

- Would paramedics be expected to 'take up the slack' left by the reduction in junior doctors hours? Would this involve more skill acquisition?

- Could paramedics be employed at the polyclinics?

- What impact would this have on the service at times of major incident?

- How many lives would be lost during transit to major A&Es? Indeed, would you even be able to get there, considering traffic and chaos during major incidents?

- If you managed to get there, would there be the staff (nurses and doctors) to whom you could hand over the patient's care?

All these questions (and more) arise from a few excerpts of an article. This demonstrates how social policy is everyone's business and how decisions made at the highest level really do have an impact on every practitioner in any healthcare setting or profession. The consultant who has written the article will obviously look at the proposed changes from his own perspective and that of his profession. Paramedics and their professional body need to be involved in social policy developments, if only to comment from their perspective. The power of professions should not be underestimated. All too often, within the health service, we are happy to have our power dispersed, in order to meet our own profession's goals. If all healthcare professions worked with a common goal and united against unpopular proposals for change, which are very often to the detriment of the patient and family, the changes may not be sanctioned. No professional can aim to achieve this unless they have a knowledge of policy documents and keep up to date with new developments.

Conclusion

An awareness of the Department of Health structure is a step towards understanding the process of policy development. The above is a working example of the role that social policy has to play in the lives of us all, in particular the lives of pre-hospital clinicians. An awareness of social policy proposals means that there is an opportunity to comment in a professional or personal capacity at the discussion stage. The results of the consultation document *Direction of Travel for Urgent Care* were due to be published, as a White Paper, in Spring 2007. As of October 2007 this has not occurred, possibly due to change of party leader and/or opposition to the reforms by local communities. Being up to date with current social policy in relation to pre-hospital care implies that clinicians are aware of what this may mean for them and colleagues in the future shape of ambulance services and has the potential to highlight areas of personal development and career opportunities.

Chapter key points

- Distinguishes between policy associated with practice and that shaping future services.
- Explains the value of understanding policy to the individual practitioner.
- Explains the role of the Department of Health in policy development and the relationship to other bodies (Strategic Health Authorities, Primary Care Trusts).
- Defines the terms White and Green Papers.
- Discusses the most relevant documents to ambulance clinician practice: *Our Health, Our Care, Our Say* (DoH 2006a); *Direction of Travel for Urgent Care* (DoH 2006d); *Emergency Access* (DoH 2006e).
- Provide a 'real' example of how the consultation documents are affecting local service provision.

References and suggested reading

British Broadcasting Corporation (2007) Hospital protest heads to London, *BBC News*. www.news.bbc.co.uk/go/pr/fr/-/1/hi/england/sussex/6225354. (Accessed 1 July 2007.)

Department of Health (2006a) *Our Health, Our Care, Our Say*. London: Stationery Office.

Department of Health (2006b) *Our Health, Our Care, Our Say: A New Direction for Community Services*. London: Stationery Office.

Department of Health (2006c) *Our Health, Our Care, Our Say: Making It Happen*. London: Stationery Office.

Department of Health (2006d) *Direction of Travel for Urgent Care: A Discussion Document*. London: Stationery Office.

Department of Health (2006e) *Emergency Access. Clinical Case for Change. Report by Sir George Alberti, the National Director for Emergency Access*. London: Stationery Office.

Ham, C. (2004) *Health Policy in Britain*, 5th edn. Basingstoke: Palgrave Macmillan.

NAO (National Audit Office) (2006) *The Provision of Out-of-Hours Care in England*. London: National Audit Office.

Nunn, D. (2007) Why Labour's new 'super surgeries' will put lives at risk, *Daily Mail*, 17 July: 50.

Peckham, S. and Meerabeau, L. (2007) *Social Policy for Nurses and the Helping Professions*, 2nd edn. Maidenhead: Open University Press/McGraw-Hill Education.

14

Leadership styles and the decision-making process
Alison Cork

Topics covered:

Introduction

This chapter is split into two sections. The first part discusses the variety of leadership styles and the work of several eminent theorists in this field. The subject of leadership is discussed in relation to the pre-hospital environment and the unique work of paramedics, where applicable and appropriate. The second part looks at the theory which lies behind the decision-making process.

Why is this relevant?

Paramedics make decisions on a daily basis. Some involve life and death decisions; others are less urgent but may still impact on the outcome for many patients and their families. The second part of this chapter explores some of the theories associated with decision making and I hope that it may impact on your future patient care.

Leadership styles and the impact on practice

Introduction

Leadership is a complex process by which a person influences others to accomplish a mission, task or objective and it is a role which is implicit in paramedic practice. From leading the coordinated approach to a multiple casualty situation to working with a colleague and assuming control of the situation, the philosophy of leadership is similar. This chapter will explore in detail the concept of leadership. By examining different models it will then concentrate on the characteristics of a good leader. Finally it will look at the requirements of a good follower, which is essential if the process is to succeed.

What constitutes a leader?

Good leaders develop through a continuous process of reflection, education and experience. However, in order to provide good leadership you must commence with the conclusion in mind in order to have a clear understanding of your destination. Leadership is a multifaceted process by which a person influences others to achieve a mission, task, or objective and directs the organization in a way that makes it more unified and consistent. Northouse (2004) argues that some people are leaders because of their formal position within an organization whereas others are leaders because of the way other group members respond to them. He describes these two types of leadership as assigned and emergent respectively. The assigned leader would be the boss. The emergent leader would be the person within the group who has the most influence, regardless of her title. Emergent leadership is acquired through other people in the organization who support and accept the person's behaviour and it is always salutary to remember that being the boss does not make you the leader; it merely gives you the power.

The work of John Adair

John Adair, a military tutor by background, developed his Action-centred Leadership model whilst lecturing at Sandhurst Royal Military Academy. He helped change the accepted perception of management to encompass leadership and has written over 25 books on the subject. He asserts that there are core functions of leadership which can be applied in any situation (Box 14.1).

Box 14.1 Core functions of leadership

Planning – seeking information, setting aims, defining tasks
Initiating – briefing, task allocation, setting standards
Controlling – maintaining standards, ensuring progress, ongoing decision making
Supporting – monitoring and rewarding individuals' contributions, encouraging team spirit, morale boosting, reconciling
Informing – clarifying tasks and plans, updating, receiving feedback and interpreting
Evaluating – feasibility of ideas, performance, enabling self-assessment

Action-centred leadership

The action–centred leadership model is a simple model which is easy to remember and straightforward to apply in clinical practice in relation to both leadership and management (Box 14.2). It is part of an integrated approach and although the three elements are collectively dependent they are also independently crucial.

Adair maintains that good leaders should have full control of the three main areas and that being able to do all these things and keep the balance right gets results by developing the team and productivity, building morale and enhancing quality, and is the mark of a successful manager and leader.

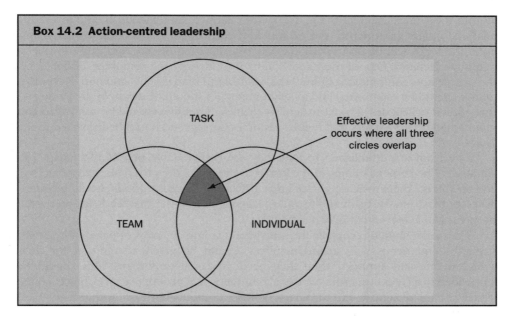

Box 14.2 Action-centred leadership

TASK

Effective leadership occurs where all three circles overlap

TEAM

INDIVIDUAL

Within each domain there are certain elements for the leader to consider and achieve (see Box 14.3).

Box 14.3 Elements which require completion

The task	Define the task
	Identify resources
	Create the plan
	Establish the responsibilities
	Set the standards
	Control and maintain the activities
	Monitor overall performance
	Review, reassess, adjust plan
	Establish standards of performance and behaviour
	Monitor and maintain discipline and integrity

The team	Resolve conflict
	Develop team working
	Encourage the team to achieve the task
	Give feedback to the group
	Understand the team members
The individual	Assist and support individuals
	Agree individual responsibilities
	Give recognition and praise
	Develop individual freedom and autonomy

Within the clinical field all the above factors happen simultaneously and are rarely analysed in any great depth. For example, when managing a multiple casualty situation the focus will be on the task, i.e. the prioritization of care and safe transfer to definitive facilities. One of the leader's aims is to identify the resources available, i.e. the people and equipment required and available to manage the situation. Responsibilities should be established and all team members should be aware of their role and that of their colleagues in order to achieve the task. Activities should be controlled and maintained by the leaders and regular reports on progress should be imparted to the team.

The team are established in that they are the available people to manage the situation. The responsibilities of the leader are to focus the group on their objectives and encourage them to achieve their aims. Effective communications should be established both within the team and to external agencies in order that feedback on overall progress and achievement may be attained.

The leader should recognize the individual variants in terms of personality, skills, strengths and needs. The team members should be given recognition for their achievements and support when they need guidance or tuition. This should be embedded in all teams in order for them to function at a productive level; however, the leader should recognize extraordinary contributions to the team and reward these appropriately.

Other models of leadership

Although within contemporary practice an authoritarian and task-led approach to leadership is sometimes utilized there are other models that incorporate the softer side of leadership which can be equally successful. One of these is the Arch of Leadership as proposed by Jooste (2004) (Box 14.4). This differs from Adair's model as she concentrates on leadership as opposed to leadership and management. Her philosophy is that there is a difference between management and leadership, which she describes as 'legitimate power and control vs empowerment and change' (Jooste 2004: 218). She asserts that the healthcare environment should move towards a scenario of more influence and less power and authority. In contemporary practice we should use influence to ensure that work, behavioural and change processes flow smoothly. Within this the capacity to motivate, persuade, appreciate, negotiate and understand are important.

Jooste (2004) proposes the arch of leadership as a model to guide the leader. This, she says, could have several uses: as a guideline for effective leadership, to examine the characteristics of an effective leader and also to identify and solve problems in the health management sector.

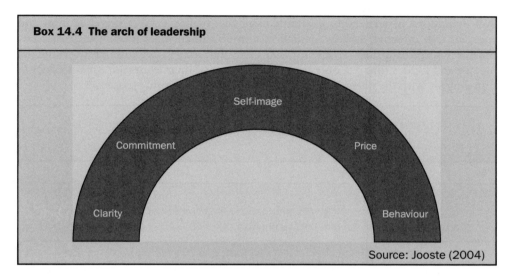

Box 14.4 The arch of leadership

Self-image

Commitment

Price

Clarity

Behaviour

Source: Jooste (2004)

To explain this model further we need to break it down into its component parts.

- Clarity – are the workers clear about their tasks? The leader should conceptualize what is right and communicate the future vision of the service to the followers. The followers should be clear about this and the time frames that are being set.
- Commitment – what do the followers need from their leaders?
- Self-image – do followers know their own abilities?
- Price – what is the price they pay or receive, financial, emotional or professional?
- Behaviour – does the leadership style promote positive and effective behaviour among followers?

Transformational leadership

The transformational approach to leadership challenges the autocratic unilateral leadership style of former years. It strives to elevate the needs of followers that are harmonious with their own goals and objectives and it achieves this through charisma, intellectual ability and individual consideration. The transformational leader is categorized as a visionary or catalyst for change that can motivate and energize staff to pursue mutual goals, share vision and create an empowering culture. With transformational leadership both the leader and the follower have the same purpose and they raise one another to higher levels of performance. It also relies on mutuality, cooperation rather than competition, networking rather than hierarchy and empowerment of all employees. Bass *et al.* cited in Murphy (2005) recognize that transformational leadership has a cascading effect and if practised at the top of the organization this has a domino effect which alters the behaviours through the lower levels. The results of such an approach are that of increased work satisfaction and a low staff turnover. Workers are more likely to stick with an organization that values their ideas and thoughts and which creates an empowering culture. Although there are more than 300 definitions of leadership currently available, Cullen (2007) urges caution and suggests that effective leaders operate in a multi-dimensional framework that combines a multitude of skills, styles, attributes and abilities. He cites numerous leaders in history and argues that it is only the effective parts of their leadership that is concentrated upon, with the narrative largely ignoring the less helpful aspects.

Stop and think – How would you describe the culture of your organization?

Links to Chapter 3 for more in-depth information about communication and Chapter 6 to explore the potential value of reflective practice.

Leadership is the style and manner in which a situation is approached. There are normally three styles and the emphasis of power is different for each one (Box 14.5).

While it is inevitable that one style will dominate behaviour, a good leader will use all three approaches and be able to alter this in any given situation. However, there are certain factors which will determine the style to be used and these are identified in Box 14.6.

Stop and think – What do you think best describes yourself? Is this how others see you?

Authoritarian

This is a style which does not look for the advice of followers, rather it is used when the leader tells the employees what they want done and how they want it done. This is most commonly used when all the information to solve the problem is available, employees are well motivated and time is of the essence. There is no room for negotiation within the decision. McCormick and Wardrope (2003) suggest that this is a style to be employed in the resuscitation situation. In this situation the leader is very much in command. From the didactic approach of resuscitation courses all members of the team will know their roles. The leader has to assess the problem quickly, work out a management plan and then give clear orders to the rest of the team. Although the leader will listen to suggestions from the members of the team, most of the direction and orders will come from the leader. Here the needs of the individual staff members are of a low priority while the key objective of saving the patient's life is paramount.

Box 14.5 Emphasis of power with different approaches

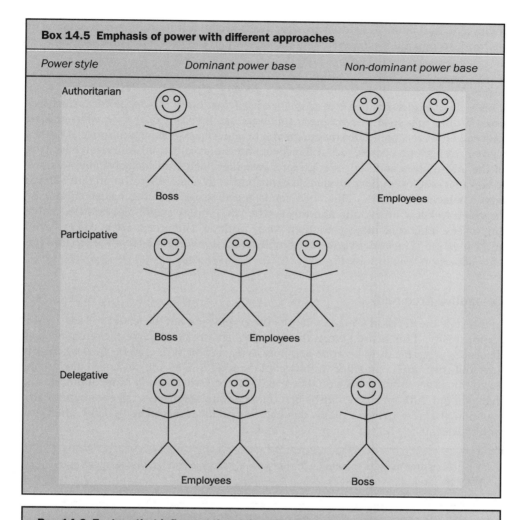

| Power style | Dominant power base | Non-dominant power base |

Authoritarian — Boss / Employees

Participative — Boss / Employees

Delegative — Employees / Boss

Box 14.6 Factors that influence the style to be used

- The resources available, i.e. time, financial, equipment
- The basis of relationships, i.e. trust, distrust
- The information holder: you, the employees, both
- The skills and knowledge of you and your employees
- Internal dynamics of the team
- Positive and negative stress levels

Although one can understand the reasons why this style is adopted in this situation the good leader will recognize that the casualty of this style of leadership is the follower. This style can be used when working with a technician who is new to the job and needs direction and firm guidance. However, it must be noted that taking such an inflexible approach does not allow the followers to develop problem-solving skills for themselves and limits individual growth; this is acceptable if, in the whole scheme of the work scenario, it is tempered with periods of participative styles of leadership.

Participative

This style of leadership involves employee participation in the decision-making process. Within this style one or more followers are involved in the decision-making process. However, the leader maintains the final decision-making authority. This is a sign of strength that employees will respect and is normally used when you have part of the information and your employees have other parts. It is inclusive and acknowledges that employees have a valuable contribution to make when shaping the service within which they work. This style sends the message that the leader cannot be expected to know everything and this is why you employ skilful and knowledgeable employees. This style may be adopted when working with an experienced crew who know their job. The leader knows the problem and the workers know their job and can offer advice on how to solve it.

Delegative (free rein)

In this style the decision is made solely by the employees, but the leader still carries the responsibility. This is used when the followers are able to analyse the situation and determine what needs to be done and how to do it. This style is to be used when you have full trust and confidence in the people around you as you cannot blame others when things go wrong. This would be used with a crew who knew more about the job than you did. Although you may be first on scene and assume overall command of the situation, if a crew arrived to assist that had been in the same situation before then you would delegate the role of leadership to them.

 Stop and think of examples in your working day where the varying styles have their uses.

It is recognized in nursing that in order for leaders to be effective the organizational culture needs to be changed (Grohar-Murray and DiCroce 2003), and a comparison can be drawn with the ambulance service. With its history steeped in military tradition the approach has been that of a goal-oriented focus which demands results. This could be said of any publicly funded organization and the reasons why are transparent; however, it is important to understand that different approaches exist and that these will produce results.

Along with the emerging styles of leadership there is an acknowledgement that the topic of followers is also worthy of further study. Hughes *et al.* (1999) cite Kelly (1988) when they agree that effective followers have the foresight to see the forest as well as the trees, the social capability to work and interact well with others, the strength of character to flourish without heroic status, and moral and psychological stability to follow corporate and personal objectives at no cost to either.

Followers will go along with the leaders for a number of differing reasons, some personal, others more objective. Some examples might be if the followers respect both the leader and the solution, if they trust the leader not to lead them into disarray, or if they like the personal characteristics of the leader. Northouse (2004) cites Blanchard *et al.* (1985), who refer to developmental levels of followers, or, as he terms it, sub-ordinates; however, it must be recognized that followers are not always subordinate to the leader. He claims that the degree to which followers have the competence and commitment necessary to accomplish a given task or activity is their developmental level. This is supported by Hughes *et al.* (1999), who state that junior followers will need almost constant guidance, coaching and comment whereas senior ones only need general guidance and periodic feedback in order to maintain high levels of performance. Moreover, they assert that the inexperienced refer to the experienced for guidance and advice on how to improve their performance. Within the framework of work-based learning for the student paramedic and technician, the student would look to the senior for guidance and feedback on performance. Although touching base with the leader periodically, i.e. the education and development centre, there is a system in which the senior follower takes on the role of leader for short periods of time. This model also helps to create new leaders as good leaders create good followers who then become good leaders, and so on. This shows that success or failure is not dependent on the leader but the followers have a role to play and this must be recognized.

Empowerment

However, the follower can only act in this way if empowered to do so. Empowerment is a term which is talked about synonymously with leadership and a good leader can be said to empower followers to be leaders of the future. Jooste (2004) recommends a number of strategies to ensure that followers recognize that they are valued and can make a positive contribution to the care of others (see Box 14.7).

Box 14.7 Strategies to develop a culture of empowerment

- Enlist others
- Strengthen others
- Foster collaboration
- Celebrate and cheer accomplishment
- Recognize contributions

This can be achieved by four simple steps in the work place (Sofarelli and Brown 1998).

1   Management of attention: employees should be aware of current objectives, events and relationships. In other words, the paramedic in clinical practice should be able not only to know the response targets for her service but also the consequences of not achieving them. She needs to understand the relationship between the target, the funding strategies, public perception of the service and the effect that it all has on staff morale.

2   Management of meaning: it is the leader's responsibility to inspire a vision to all employees. A good leader will acknowledge the problems within the service and not exist in utopia but suggest ways in which small changes can have large impacts.

3   Management of trust: leader and follower must trust each other to facilitate empowerment. This is one of the most important aspects of empowerment. The follower has to be assured that the leader is in control and can determine the outcome in a positive light.

4   Management of self: high self-awareness, self-regard and self-esteem. This could be one of the more difficult aspects of empowerment. This can be best explored by describing disempowerment as a state in which individuals are deprived of opportunities for growth and development. They are excluded from the decision-making process and frequently lack resources to do their job properly. Murphy (2005) considers that the consequence of this is that they feel frustrated, incompetent and have little loyalty to the organization. In order to create a culture of empowerment this is usually the first objective that has to be addressed.

Theories of decision making

Introduction

Ambulance clinicians make decisions every day while planning and delivering care within their scope of practice. Successful and reliable decision making requires the attainment and utilization of relevant data as well as higher order thinking skills such as decision making and critical thinking. This chapter will explore the theory of decision making and relate it to the paramedic's practice.

What is decision making?

Effective decision making is a pivotal role in the delivery of quality care and the advancement of clinical services. It is a process which happens with every episode of patient contact, although the progression of the decision is rarely analysed in any depth. Not only should reflection occur when decisions go wrong but also when they are successful decisions. It is often the case that the successful outcome is not reviewed in any depth, thereby denying the learning process that could accompany it.

Link to Chapter 6 for examples of models of reflection.

By following a decision-making model it enables the component parts of any action to be analysed and the weakness or strength of the decision-making process recognized. However, decisions in clinical practice rarely follow a linear logical pattern.

Intertwined with clinical decision making is that of problem solving and these two concepts are often used interchangeably, though there are subtle differences. Decision making is where alternative courses of action are judged on their merits and only one of these is ultimately selected whereas problem solving is a process in which a dilemma, once analysed, is identified and the cause then corrected. It encompasses the decision-making process, which is said to be synonymous with management and is one of the criteria on which management expertise is judged. Problem solving is a systematic process that focuses on analysing a difficult situation; considerable time and energy is spent on identifying the real problem and it can be described as the precursor to decision making. In practice, however, it is sometimes difficult to separate the two, e.g. the paramedic dealing with a violent patient might choose not to solve the root cause of the violent conduct, such as personality trait, alcohol or drug intoxication or dependence. As an alternative he may choose to utilize only decision-making skills to call for police assistance to facilitate removal of the patient to police custody. The paramedic has, therefore, made the decision to remove the problem, i.e. the violent patient, rather than examine the cause of the patient's behaviour and address that. This is not opting out of the situation; rather it is identifying the resources available and utilizing them to best advantage.

What can help us make decisions?

Decision making exists within a framework of classifications. Routine decisions are those that are made when the problem is well defined and commonplace in practice. There are usually established policies and procedures which can be used to guide decision makers as the problem has been examined and solved by previous practitioners before them. In contrast, adaptive decisions are where problems and alternative solutions are somewhat unusual and only partially understood. There may be a policy to support the decision-making process but as the problem and solution is ill defined, creative thought may be necessary. The last area is that of innovative decisions. This is when the problem is unusual and unclear and in order to make a decision creative thinking and innovative solutions are necessary (Sullivan and Decker 2005). An example of this would be referring a patient with a mental health problem directly to her community psychiatric nurse rather than her general practitioner because of the patient's preference. This decision would circumnavigate the accepted practice of contacting the general practitioner but would be more individualized for the patient. Within emergency work there are routine decisions that fall within policy and procedures, but there may be the need for innovative decisions if the patient's situation warrants it. It is then that an understanding of the decision-making process will be invaluable to guide the paramedic to the best course of action.

 Stop and think – What enables you to make decisions? Think of an example where you may not have agreed with policy and procedures. What difference may it have made to a patient outcome?

Decision making is a complex cognitive process that is defined as choosing a particular course of action, implying that there are several courses of action that could be taken and that a considered judgement is required to decide which route to follow.

Inherent within decision making is the concept of critical thinking. This is purposeful, goal-orientated thinking that is based on a body of knowledge which is derived from research and other sources of authenticated evidence (Ignatavicius 2001). It is more complex than problem solving and decision making because it involves a higher level of reasoning and deductive thinking.

Critical thinking

Decision making relies heavily on critical thinking skills. These are described as the process of probing underlying assumptions, interpreting and evaluating arguments, imagining and exploring alternatives and developing a sense of reflective criticism (Sullivan and Decker 2005). These are integral to effective practice and are described in Box 14.8.

Box 14.8 Critical thinking skills

Interpretation – clarifying data
Analysis – understanding data
Evaluation – determining outcome
Inference – drawing conclusions
Explanation – justifying actions based on data
Self-regulation – examining one's own practice

(Ignatavicius 2001)

There are certain qualities that successful decision makers will possess. They have to have the willingness to take a risk, the sensitivity to react both to the situation and to the other members involved in the decision-making process, the energy to make things happen and the creativity to develop new ways to solve problems. Such people have a lot of balls to juggle, as represented in figure 14.1, but they do possess a repertoire of skills that they can call on to assist them in the decision-making process.

 Stop and think – Is critical thinking encouraged in your organization?

 Stop and think – Do you possess any of the traits of a critical thinker? How might your personality traits make your working life more frustrating, if you feel constrained by your organization's policies/procedures?

With any decision there are individual variations which may affect the outcomes. Any choices generated and made are affected by personal values. These are moral and ethical codes socialized within us as part of our culture, exposure and experience.

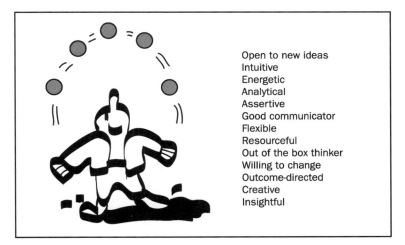

Figure 14.1 Characteristics of a critical thinker
Source: Marquis and Huston (2006)

These could be those that have been instilled in us as children or those values that we have acquired through our workplace culture and customs. These values are also imposed upon us by the changing society that we live in. In our current climate the paramedic who goes into a patient's house when a relative is smoking may make the decision to ask the relative to put the cigarette out or leave the room. This is in response to society's anxieties about the effects of passive smoking. This may not have been a problem in the 1970s when smoking was more accepted by society. Although at times biases will be acknowledged and addressed within the decision-making process there will also be times when the value is so implicit that it is not obvious.

Link to Chapter 11 to read about the process of socialization and factors that influence who we are.

The value of experience

Within the process of decision making we use our life experiences to guide the way in which we act. Cioffi (1997) defines this as intuitive knowing associated with past personal experiences, which she refers to as heuristics in her literature. The more mature a person the greater range of alternatives he may identify. This may not be maturity in the traditional meaning of age but of time spent in his chosen career. The effect of past experiences and outcomes all guide us to make certain decisions as we draw on these to guide our thinking. There are those, however, who do not re-examine decisions that they have made and therefore do not learn from their experiences. It is always advisable to remember that we do not learn by doing, rather we learn by doing and then reviewing. Cioffi (1997) states that intuitive, heuristic judgements are qualitative, critical, discriminating and associated with past experiences and she identifies six key aspects of heuristic decision making, maintaining that they can be used in complex decision-making situations (see Box 14.9).

Box 14.9 Heuristic decision making

Pattern recognition – recognition of patterns of responses presented by patients

Similarity recognition – comparison of similar and dissimilar characteristics of past patients who have had similar conditions

Common-sense understanding – understanding diversity from a selection of information, i.e. vital signs that give subtle trends/indications about a patient

Skilled knowhow – that considers possibilities for each patient

Sense of salience – perceptions about a patient that stand out as more important

Deliberative rationality – selective attention of certain aspects/events

(Cioffi 1997: 205)

Models of decision making

In order to support the decision-making process various models are available and within the process there are critical elements that determine outcome. These are described as follows:

- Determine the goal
- Gather data carefully
- Generate many alternatives
- Think logically
- Choose and act decisively

Carroll and Johnson (1990), cited in Muir (2004), suggest a seven-step model which incorporates recognizing the situation, generating alternatives and clarifying choices, as outlined in Box 14.10.

Box 14.10 Decision-making model

1. Recognition of the situation
2. Formulation of an explanation
3. Alternative generation of other explanations
4. Information search to clarify choices and available evidence
5. Judgement or choice
6. Action
7. Feedback

(Carroll and Johnson 1990)

In comparison to Carroll and Johnson (1990), Marquis and Huston (2006) describe a model commonly applied to healthcare situations (Box 14.11). Following a similar strategy to Carroll and Johnson (1990) they use slightly different terms, although the philosophy is the same.

Box 14.11 Traditional problem-solving model

1.   Identify the problem

2.   Gather data to analyse the causes and consequences

3.   Explore the alternatives

4.   Evaluate the alternatives

5.   Select the appropriate solution

6.   Implement the solution

7.   Evaluate the results

(Marquis and Huston 2006)

With the above model, Marquis and Huston (2006) recognize that the decision-making process does not take place until step 5. They also state that the weakness of this model lies in the amount of time needed for proper implementation and the lack of initial objective setting.

Within the climate in which the paramedic currently works there are numerous opportunities for barriers to effective decision making to exist. These reflect closely the barriers that are discussed in relation to change management.

Link to Chapter 15 for more detail on change management.

Barriers to decision making

Barriers may exist at both an operational and an organizational level. At an organizational level there can be a lack of managers who have been adequately prepared to take on the role of decision makers (Finkelman 2006). They may lack the skills to communicate effectively with their teams in order to promote the message of the decision that has been made. A lack of staff participation will effectively immobilize the decision as it should include all stakeholders, a huge although not unachievable task when examining the ambulance clinician provision within the United Kingdom. At a more local operational level one of the main barriers is that of taking shortcuts within the process (Sullivan and Decker 2005). This can limit the amount of data collection and the quantity and quality of the alternatives that are generated and then considered.

Link to Chapter 3 to explore the value of communication and barriers to effective communication and Chapter 4, pages 43–8, for further explanation of the clinical audit process.

A barrier which straddles both organizational and operational levels is that of rigid ideas and points of view. If the stakeholders do not want to embrace the decision because of preconceived ideas or past experiences the decision maker will have to ensure that these views are discussed and new ways forward negotiated. This will be demonstrated in the clinical setting with phrases such as 'We have always done it this way; it did not work when we tried to change it before; it is easier to keep it as it is.' It must be recognized by the decision maker that the opposition is ignored at the peril of the decision being unsuccessful.

At a more individual level, the personality trait of the decision maker can act as a barrier. One's personality can and does affect the decision-making process. The decision making could be based on approval seeking if the manager is inexperienced and seeking acceptance from the workers. Rather than face rejection, when a truly difficult decision arises the manager will make a decision which is based on the fact that it will placate people, so increasing the manager's popularity. Alternatively, a manager may make a decision based on her own personality traits, rather than that of her workers. The 'workaholic' boss may deem it acceptable to ask the staff to work overtime without payment if this is what she herself would do. This is a common pitfall of managers and they must work hard to embrace all personality types into the team and not judge others by their own standards if these are not the norm.

 Stop and think – Do any of the above comments have resonance to you?

The second part of this chapter has demonstrated that with any decision made in practice there should be a process of reflection afterwards. Decisions are made all the time in clinical practice but are rarely reflected upon unless something untoward happens. It is important to be aware of the barriers to effective decision making in order to reduce these, or at least acknowledge that they exist and can affect the outcome. In order to ensure that decisions made are effective, the process of following a model will enable logical analysis to be applied.

Conclusion

Overall this chapter has demonstrated that leadership and decision-making skills are not in addition to, but part of, the clinical repertoire that enables effective skilled care to be delivered to the patient. Although not obvious at the point of care delivery, an understanding of the ways in which leadership and decision making are approached will develop an understanding of the wider issues of working within the organization.

Chapter key points

- Being the boss does not make you the leader; it merely gives you the power.
- Leadership does not have to be on a large scale; rather it can be on a job-to-job basis.
- Understanding the component parts of the decision-making process enables a higher level of reflection.

References and suggested reading

Adair, J. (1988) *The Action-centred Leader*. London: Kogan Page.

Carroll, J. and Johnson, E. (1990) *Decision Research: A Field Guide*. Thousand Oaks, CA: Sage Publications.

Cioffi, J. (1997) Heuristics, servants to intuition, in clinical decision-making, *Journal of Advanced Nursing*, 26(1): 203–8.

Cullen, J. (2007) Front line leadership: a challenge to the continual search for the holy grail of an all-encompassing leadership model, *Leadership in Public Services*, 3(1): 4–16.

Finkelman, A. (2006) *Leadership and Management in Nursing*. London: Prentice-Hall.

Grohar-Murray, M. and DiCroce, H. (2003) *Leadership and Management in Nursing*, 3rd edn. London: Prentice-Hall.

Hughes, R., Ginnett, R. and Curphy, G. (1999) *Leadership: Enhancing the Lessons of Experience*. London: McGraw-Hill.

Ignatavicius, D. (2001) Critical thinking skills for the bedside nurse, *Nursing Management*, 32(1): 37–9.

Jooste, K. (2004) Leadership: a new perspective, *Journal of Nursing Management*, 12: 217–23.

McCormick, S. and Wardrope, J. (2003) Major incidents, leadership, and series summary review, *Emergency Medicine Journal*, 20: 70–4.

Marquis, B. and Huston, C. (2006) *Leadership Roles and Management Functions in Nursing*, 5th edn. Philadelphia, PA: Lippincott Williams and Wilkins.

Marriner Tomey, A. (2004) *Guide to Nursing Management and Leadership*, 7th edn. St. Louis, MI: Mosby.

Muir, N. (2004) Clinical decision-making: theory and practice, *Nursing Standard*, 18(36): 47–52.

Murphy, L. (2005) Transformational leadership: a cascading chain reaction, *Journal of Nursing Management*, 12: 128–36.

Northouse, P. (2004) *Leadership Theory and Practice*, 3rd edn. London: Sage Publications.

Sofarelli, D. and Brown, D. (1998) The need for nursing leadership in uncertain times, *Journal of Nursing Management*, 6: 201–7.

Sullivan, E. and Decker, P. (2005) *Effective Leadership and Management in Nursing*. London: Prentice-Hall.

15

Change management theory and its usefulness to practice
Alison Cork

Topics covered:

- Introduction
- Why is this relevant?
- Supporting change
- Strategies for managing change
- The change agent
- Improving patient care
- Change models
- Conclusion
- Chapter key points
- References and suggested reading

Introduction

This chapter aims to explore the main theories of change management. It will explore barriers to change and how these can be overcome.

Why is this relevant?

One of the main challenges for today's practitioners is to keep abreast of current clinical, educational, political and local changes that affect everyday practice within the wider NHS and its local providers. Change is inevitable within any organization; the sheer size of the NHS and the influence of five-year electoral cycles means that the NHS experiences more change than most organizations. The skill of change management can be learnt and can be a positive, motivating and empowering experience, but so often NHS employees experience negative, demotivating and demoralizing changes. Clinicians who understand change management are more likely to be able to influence change in a positive manner, creating an empowered workforce which can only be positive for patient care.

Supporting change

In order to deliver a first class service we continually need to examine what we are doing and question whether there is a need to change our practices. Change happens at a multitude of levels: as an organizational approach, at an operational level or as a personal achievement. This is how the NHS has evolved from its initial stages of being a system which delivered health care in a paternalistic fashion into what we now recognize to be a partnership in care between the clinician and the patient. We also have to recognize that, as the health service has evolved, so has society. For instance, patients' expectations are far greater in the modern healthcare system than has traditionally been experienced. With the emergence of the multi-faceted media, patients now have access to the most up-to-date information, treatment and research regarding their disease/condition and so are better informed.

In order to deliver care that is based on contemporary evidence we need to ensure that the climate within which we work is one that is conducive to change. Finkelman (2006) considers the climate required for change and discusses a state she terms 'readiness for change'. She further defines this as being willing to take on the challenge of change and invest in the effort that it requires. She claims that this is affected by trust and that the relationship between staff and management is pivotal to the success of the change. Within the relationship the manager has to be open to new ideas engendered by the staff, recognizing that all of the participants have an important role to play in the process.

Strategies for managing change

There are several strategies that have been identified for managing change and the approach taken will depend upon the type of change that is to be effected.

Power–coercive strategies

These are based on the application of power by legitimate authority, economic sanctions or political influence. Within this strategy changes are made through law, policy or financial appropriations. There is a penalty, be it financial or political, for not enforcing the changes and those that are in power may be unable to stop this. These strategies involve the compliance of less powerful people with the leadership, plans and directions of more powerful individuals. They acknowledge the need to use sources of power to bring about change and do not deny the intelligence and rationality of people or the importance of their values and beliefs: an example of this would be a change of policy. This is the type of change that is so often faced within the ambulance service and the health service as a whole, in which the individual has little or no power or input to the change and is expected to conform or face penalties. An example of this would be the ambulance response times that are monitored and then used as a quality mechanism to judge performance.

Empirical–rational strategies

The empirical–rational strategy is based on the assumption that people are rational and will act according to logical self-interest. It assumes that if a change has been shown to be justified and the individual concerned can benefit from it then he will be more willing to adopt such a change. Within this strategy, knowledge is the key. It is assumed that the change agent who has the knowledge also has the expert power to persuade people to accept a rationally justified change that will benefit them. Sullivan and Decker (2005) describe the flow of influence as moving from those who know to those who do not know. This assumes that the expert is the change agent and is involved in the application of the change rather than facilitating others to introduce new ideas. An example of this could be changing practice on a small scale between two practitioners, where one would be the expert and the other the participant, such as a paramedic teaching a technician or a student paramedic a new skill.

Normative–re-educative strategies

If the power–coercive strategy is the authoritarian approach then the normative–re-educative strategy is the democratic. This approach encompasses the feeling side of change. It assumes that people act in accordance with social norms and values. The change agent using this type of approach must focus on the roles, attitudes and feelings of the stakeholders, as this will influence their acceptance of the change. The challenge for change agents in this approach is not to use power, but rather their interpersonal skills of collaboration and negotiation in order to effect change. This approach is very well suited to the problem solving needed in health care today and can be used in a variety of ways, such as determining and delivering health promotion needs of patients.

The change agent

The pivotal area of success is that of the change agent, her influence upon the process and the characteristics she possesses (see Box 15.1). Marquis and Huston (2006) assert that a change agent is a person skilled in the theory and implementation of a planned change. Huczynski and Buchanan (2001) expand on this theme and claim that the change agent seems to require fewer technical skills and more interpersonal and managerial skills in communication, presentation, negotiation and influencing and selling.

Box 15.1 Characteristics of a successful change agent

- Experience both of change and of the service undergoing the change
- Success at work
- Being respected by the team
- Proven leadership skills
- Management competencies

(Grohar-Murray and DiCroce 2003: 265)

Although the change agent may be the person who has the vision, he needs to recognize that it is the participants in the process who will determine whether the change is successful. In order to be successful, the change agent has to have influence and Sullivan (2004) states that this is more important than authority when looking at change. She advises that it is wise to use influence before authority when trying to implement new ways of working or any other kind of change and she defines influence as to the extent to which one can communicate ideas to others and gain their support through participation or acceptance. Given Sullivan's (2004) reference to authority and power it follows on that change agents should be considered at all levels. Change is often seen as a big deal and one which utilizes extensive resources; however, practitioners need to be aware that they can effect change in their immediate working environment by adopting some of the characteristics of the ideal change agent and encouraging colleagues to think about alternative ways of working.

The change agent's main responsibility is to manage the situation by developing a plan. This should include a description of the change and the rationale for it; the objectives should be set in measurable terms and the projected timetable should be included. The plan should be transparent and available for all involved to view. Secrecy surrounding change engenders feelings of distrust and insecurity, thereby reducing the chance of success.

The change agent needs to be someone with the drive and enthusiasm to support the change when it is flagging and to convince others that the change is achievable. With this in mind it is obvious that the change agent is required to have complete faith in the success of the change at its fruition.

With any planned change some preparatory work needs to be undertaken in order to predict the relative success of that change (Tiffany and Lutjens 1998). People will respond to change in a number of ways and those who may not embrace the change at the outset may be the greatest supporters at its conclusion. Regardless of the type of change it all brings feelings of achievement, loss, pride and stress to the fore (Marquis and Huston 2006). If the change agent is to be successful the different behaviours and responses need to be managed in a supportive manner. Huczynski and Buchanan (2001) claim that if the responses can be anticipated then knowledge should be used both to develop support for the change and to address resistance at an early stage. One of the techniques that are commonly recommended to identify the supporters and resistors of change is that of a force field analysis based on the work of Kurt Lewin (1951).

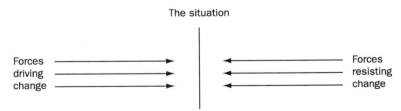

Figure 15.1 Force field analysis

This format shows how the driving and resisting forces oppose each other and in the present state they are equally balanced and level. In order to achieve change, first an imbalance must occur, an increase in either force, which unfreezes the present behaviour and unsettles the status quo.

Lewin (1951) proposes that when implementing any change there are a number of factors that help to achieve change (drivers) as well as factors that may impede change (resistors). He further argues that it is easier to remove the resisting forces than it is to generate new driving forces as the resisting forces will only increase in strength to compensate. Cork (2005) cogently argues that when using this format it is possible to conceptualize the drivers and resistors and to consider ways in which these can be diminished in a given situation.

Improving patient care

Within health care one of the focal and most persuasive drivers in order to effect any change has to be the argument of improved patient care. With any change the impact of it on the patient must be considered; however, it could be viewed as paternalistic for a body of 'experts' to decide what impact the change will have upon the patient. One of the ways to overcome this is to involve the patient at the earliest stage and this has been embraced in recent years by the Department of Health with multiple initiatives to develop a stronger local voice in the development of health and social care services (DoH 2006). Other drivers which can be used to generate support for the change include financial gain, better working conditions, increased productivity, and increased kudos to name but a few. The change agent must recognize that in order for a change to have the maximum chance of success positive drivers need to be reinforced at regular intervals.

In contrast to drivers, the resistors are people who are unable or unwilling to discuss or accept changes that are in some way damaging or threatening to the individual (Huczynski and Buchanan 2001). They emphasize that any change means discontinuity and the breakdown of familiar structures and relationships. This can be unsettling for a number of reasons: fear of the unknown, disruption of the status quo, uncertainty about new pressures or expectations on the individual, for example. Finkelman (2006) agrees with this viewpoint and adds that when there is little time for adjustment the resistance to change is greater. Sullivan and Decker (2005) provide us with some statements that resistors may use (Box 15.2).

Box 15.2 Statements that people will use that illustrate individuals' resistance to change

- We tried that before
- It won't work
- No one else does it like that
- We've always done it that way
- We can't afford it
- We do not have the time
- It will cause too much commotion

(Sullivan and Decker 2005)

Resistance is to be expected and may not always be as overt as this. There may be resistors who are working to undermine the change in a covert manner, surreptitiously undermining the efforts of the change agent. Although these are the major strategies to block change you might encounter, they are not exhaustive. A further range of behaviours is demonstrated in Box 15.3.

Box 15.3 Common responders and responses to change

- Innovators: enthusiastic and thrive on change
- Early adopters: open and receptive to new ideas
- Early majority: adopt new ideas before the average person
- Late majority: sceptical of innovation and change
- Laggards: dedicated to tradition and last to adopt a change
- Rejecters: openly oppose innovation and encourage others to oppose change also.

(Bushy and Kamphuis 1993)

Pearcey and Draper (1996) maintain that much of the resistance to change in the NHS may be due to its top-down approach. It must be questioned why, when a change is necessary, it is usually imposed from the top down rather than engendered from the bottom up. The challenge is to work with the resistors and the person who has the vision to combine this with the discontentment that may exist in order for people to appreciate the impact of the change for the individuals concerned, be they patients or colleagues. It is recognized that the greatest influence is achieved when members discuss issues that are perceived as important and make relevant and binding decisions based on those discussions. Change would be far more productive if were inclusive and representative of all the stakeholders' views.

A current example of the imposition of top-down change is the continuing prevalence of methicillin resistant staphylococcus aureus (MRSA) in our NHS Trusts. The following press extract exemplifies the fact that resistance to change clearly has the potential to affect patient care.

Quarter of NHS trusts miss targets for superbug

One in four NHS trusts in England admit they are failing to comply with hygiene regulations introduced last year to halt the spread of MRSA and other hospital superbugs, health inspectors disclose today.

The Healthcare Commission said 99 of the 394 trusts confessed to not meeting all the standards included in a compulsory hygiene code introduced by health ministers last October.

Norman Lamb, the Liberal Democrat health spokesman, said: 'It is wholly unacceptable that one in four hospitals are still failing to meet required hygiene standards . . . It is shocking that after countless government initiatives the number of hospitals failing to protect patients from these infections has doubled. Hospital staff should treat failure to comply with hygiene standards as a very serious issue, akin to gross misconduct.'

The commission said 14 per cent of trust boards were unable to sign a declaration that they 'keep patients, staff and visitors safe with systems to ensure risk of healthcare-acquired infection to patients is reduced', a failure rate almost double the percentage in last year's return.

Anna Walker, the commission's chief executive, said the apparent deterioration did not imply that the NHS was becoming less safe for patients.

The standards were included in a hygiene code imposing 11 compulsory duties on trusts to prevent the spread of infection. This concentrated the minds of trust directors and may have made many realize their systems were not as secure as had previously been thought.

(Carvel 2007)

This extract demonstrates that resistance to change is a very real threat to patient care and the achievement of government targets. Having an understanding of change theory, and understanding why people often resist change, may improve involvement in the change and subsequently reduce resistance. It could also be argued that this resistance to comply with 'top-down' directives is also due to poor leadership and managerial style. Change models can provide a useful structure for those planning change, on both a small and large scale.

Link to Chapter 14 for the theories of leadership and decision making.

Change models

There are several change models which exist and can be applied to the healthcare setting (see Box 15.4), but only Lewin (1951) will be discussed in detail. This list is not exhaustive and a prudent change agent should be aware that different models are more appropriate in relation to the main focus of the change.

Once a decision has been reached to implement a change there must be time allocated to the sequence of stages designed to reduce resistance and maintain support for others. Three familiar stages based on the work of Lewin (1951) in implementing change are:

1   unfreezing
2   moving
3   refreezing

1 Unfreeze the current situation

Lewin (1951) suggests that in this stage the current situation needs to be analysed and the need for change identified. Participants should be motivated to get ready for the change and trust needs to be built between them and the change agent. At this time

Box 15.4 Comparison of change models	
Lewin	1 unfreezing 2 moving 3 refreezing
Lippitt	1 diagnose problem 2 assess motivation 3 assess change agent's motivations and resources 4 select progressive change objects 5 choose change agent role 6 maintain change 7 terminate helping relationships
Havelock	1 building a relationship 2 diagnosing the problem 3 acquiring resources 4 choosing the solution 5 gaining acceptance 6 stabilization and self-renewal
Rogers	1 knowledge 2 persuasion 3 decision 4 implementation 5 confirmation

(Sullivan and Decker 2005: 219)

attitudes should be addressed in a non-confrontational manner and alternatives explored. It is important to ensure that adequate time is set aside for the introduction of new ideas and this should be gradual, so as not to overwhelm the individuals involved. This is a time for giving information by the change agent and this should include the reasons why a change is required and how the organization and individuals will benefit from it. The change agent should not attempt to coerce the people involved by presenting a positive stance toward the proposed change; rather, there should be honesty about temporary or permanent inconvenience in order to give the workers some sense of control. People's discomfort should be acknowledged as this will preserve everyone's dignity in the future. The change agent should recognize that change is threatening to some staff and therefore negative reactions are commonplace, but if handled in the correct manner can become positive factors in the future. It is at this time that commending the valuable ideas put forward by the staff will encourage wider constructive feedback in the future.

2 Moving

It should be at this stage that the issue or problem is clearly identified. The individuals should agree that the status quo is not beneficial to them. This could be for a number of reasons but will usually reflect the changing clinical and political climate that we currently work in. They should have a realization that to maintain the status quo will have negative consequences that can be avoided by the change process. The participants should be encouraged to view the problem from alternative perspectives, promoting a wider viewpoint than their immediate work environment in order to understand the systems which surround them. Goals and objectives are developed and strategies implemented as this is the working stage of the process where new beliefs, attitudes and ideals are promoted. It is at this transitional stage that the participants need to know exactly what is expected of them and how it contributes to the new system. This will help to reduce the ambiguity and insecurity that will accompany the uncertainty.

3 Refreezing

This is the last step of the change process but is pivotal to its success. Its goal is to prevent a return to the past. At this time there has to be reliable confirmation that the new practice is stabilized, integrated into practice and accepted by the staff. It is at this stage that it is easy to slip back to the way things were, so destabilizing the whole process. If the staff are ready to accept that change is part of the work agenda and its environment and that it serves to improve quality of care then it is far more likely to succeed. The change needs to be evaluated through ongoing monitoring processes and the change agent should be prepared to review the goal of the change and whether it is still appropriate or obtainable. Within the current climate of care delivery, however, it is often true that as one change is refreezing another is in the unfreezing change. This serves to overwhelm the participants with change and does not allow them to reorientate themselves to the current climate. A force field analysis should again be conducted in this stage to help maintain the new equilibrium until the change is embedded into accepted practice.

Link to Chapter 4, pages 44–8, for details on evaluating practice via audit.

Conclusion

As healthcare professionals working within the ambulance service it is important that you are aware of the theory that underpins any change. By understanding the relevant stages of the models and recognizing the pitfalls and barriers to successful change you can anticipate the success of any change that may be imposed upon or initiated by you. It is important to recognize that change can exist on a variety of levels, from the power coercive changes instituted by employers as a response to policy changes at a higher level or the changes that happen at station level instituted in a more democratic way to the individual changes that you will make to your own practice as a response to your ongoing learning and experience.

Chapter key points

- In order to meet the demands of our patients and evolving health care of the twenty-first century we need to be ready and willing to change.

- There are several change strategies that can be used depending on the change required.

- The key characteristics of the change agent, the importance of recognizing and managing resistors is explained.

- The importance of using change and change theory to improve patient care is discussed.

- Various change models are discussed and compared.

References and suggested reading

Bushy, A. and Kamphuis, J. (1993) Response to innovation: behavioural patterns, *Nursing Management*, 24 (3): 62–4.

Carvel, J. (2007) Quarter of NHS trusts miss targets for superbug, *Guardian*, 18 June. www.guardian.co.uk/print/0,,330041729-117700,00.html. (Accessed 2 July 2007.)

Cork, A. (2005) A model for successful change management, *Nursing Standard*, 19(25): 40–2.

Cullen, J. (2007) Front line leadership – a challenge to the continual search for the holy grail of an all-encompassing leadership model, *Leadership in Public Services*, 3(1): 4–16.

DoH (Department of Health) (2006) *Our Health, Our Care, Our Say: A New Direction for Community Services*. London: The Stationery Office.

Finkelman, A. (2006) *Leadership and Management in Nursing*. New Jersey, NJ: Pearson Prentice-Hall.

Grohar-Murray, M. and DiCroce, H. (2003) *Leadership and Management in Nursing*, 3rd edn. London: Pearson/Prentice-Hall.

Huczynski, A. and Buchanan, D. (2001) *Organizational Behaviour: An Introductory Text*, 4th edn. London: Prentice-Hall.

Lewin, K. (1951) *Field Theory in Social Science*. New York: Greenwood Press.

Marquis, B. and Huston, C. (2006) *Leadership Roles and Management Functions in Nursing*, 5th edn. Philadelphia, PA: Lippincott Williams and Wilkins.

Pearcey, P. and Draper, P. (1996) using the diffusion of innovation model to influence practice: a case study, *Journal of Advanced Nursing*, 23(4): 714–21.

Sullivan, E. (2004) *Becoming Influential: A Guide for Nurses*. London: Pearson/Prentice-Hall.

Sullivan, E. and Decker, P. (2005) *Effective Leadership and Management in Nursing*, 4th edn. Harlow: Addison-Wesley.

Tiffany, C. and Lutjens, L. (1998) *Planned Change Theories for Nursing*. London: Routledge.

16

Continuing professional development: who needs it?
Bob Fellows

Topics covered:

- Introduction
- Why is this relevant?
- The role of the HPC register
- What is continuing professional development (CPD)?
- Why do I need to record my CPD?
- Standards for CPD
- The purpose of each part of the profile
- Explanation of how HPC standards 1–5 can be demonstrated within your CPD profile
- What happens to your completed CPD profile?
- Conclusion
- Chapter key points
- References, suggested reading and useful websites

Introduction

When I joined the London Ambulance Service in 1980 I completed the six-week 'Millar course' and passed the examinations both theory and practical and, once posted to operations, applied to get on to an Intubation and Infusion (I & I) course. This I achieved in 1984 although many others testified to being on the waiting list for six to seven years. I was also expected to attend a two-week post-proficiency training course every five years. This was a programme I was never selected for as a student although I did get to teach on several when I was promoted as a young training officer. The exigencies of the ambulance service precluded me and many, many others like me from getting anywhere near a classroom as an ambulance driver/attendant and so development was down to the individual to buy a book (usually *Nancy Caroline's Emergency Care in the Street*), subscribe to a magazine (*Journal of Emergency Medical*

Services) or trek up the M1 every summer to attend Ambex (the annual exhibition and conference of the Ambulance Service Association) and listen to some of the lectures, although they were very rarely anything to do with clinical development, tending to be dominated by a managerial and political agenda that baffled me then and occasionally still does.

So, of course, development was a hit and miss affair. Did I get developed? Yes, of course, but more by my own enthusiasm and some luck than any real plan of action by the NHS or by my employer.

While writing this chapter I received a letter from the Health Professions Council which enclosed a re-registration form for me to complete and sign. This required me to declare that I was wishing to remain on the register and state that I am fit and well and that we are continuing in safe and effective practice. There was also a requirement for me to declare that I was maintaining my continuing professional development. It also reminded me that from 2008 a sample of every registrant will be looked at for compliance. In reality that meant that when I re-registered in 2009 as a paramedic I might be one of the 2.5 per cent (around 110) of paramedics audited for their CPD by HPC-appointed assessors.

Why is this relevant?

Ambulance clinicians need an understanding of their professional roles and responsibilities in relation to their governing body. This also incorporates their responsibilities pertaining to continuing professional development and their continuing registration.

The role of the HPC register

If you use a protected title (paramedic) then you will need to be on the HPC Register. Bear in mind that if you come off the register you will not be able to use the paramedic title to refer to yourself or to your work. You should also consider that you may need to update your skills to come back onto the register at a future date. To stay registered you will need to ensure that you can sign the professional declaration on your renewal form stating that you continue to meet all the standards required of you. If you are working in education, management or research, this still counts as practising your profession.

If you have moved to a non-clinical area of work but wish to stay on the register, you need to ensure that you keep up to date with your profession and that you stay within your scope of practice. And if you return to clinical work or change your scope of practice then you may need to update your skills.

When you are planning or undertaking your CPD you will need to make sure that it is relevant to your work. Similarly, to stay registered, you need to make sure you keep within the 'scope of your practice'. This refers to the particular area in which you are trained to practise, lawfully safely and effectively in a way that meets the HPC standards and does not present any risk to the patients, public or to yourself. Scope of practice may vary between paramedics and will relate to job role, experience and training. For example, two paramedics will both meet the HPCs (2003a) Standards of Proficiency (SOP), but may then have gone on to specialize in different areas. If they were then to perform each other's jobs without training, they may be practising outside their scope of practice, as their lack of experience in the different area may lead to unsafe practice, or pose a risk to a patient or to themselves.

The SOP are the standards which every registrant must meet in order to become registered and must continue to meet in order to stay on the register. They set out the required knowledge, understanding and skills for the practice of each profession. Registrants must also read and agree to abide by the Standards of Conduct, Performance and Ethics (HPC 2003b).

If someone is no longer fit to practise their profession and does not remove themselves voluntarily, the HPC can take action using the fitness to practise process. If you feel that for any reason you no longer meet these standards (of proficiency, or of conduct, performance and health) then you should come off the register. This is known as professional self-regulation; it basically means that you (the registrant) are in the best position to judge your ability to practise safely and lawfully. It is your responsibility to stay on the register, or to decide if you need to come off for any reason. Likewise, you need to inform the HPC of any changes in your circumstances which may affect your ability to practise safely. It is felt that as an accountable registered professional, you are in the best position to make professional judgements of this nature and the HPC trusts you to do so (HPC 2003b).

What is CPD?

The HPC in 2002 defined CPD as 'a range of learning activities through which health professionals maintain and develop throughout their career to ensure that they retain their capacity to practise safely, effectively and legally within their evolving scope of practice' (cited in HPC 2006: 1).

Put simply, CPD is the way paramedics continue to learn and develop throughout their careers so they keep their skills and knowledge up to date and are able to work safely, legally and effectively.

Why do I need to record my CPD?

In addition to being linked to your HPC registration, CPD is an essential part of your development as a professional. You may feel as though *recording* your CPD is not as valuable as *doing* your CPD in the first place. However, without the evidence of the value of your CPD, how will you be able to show it really was worthwhile to your service? If you don't have an up-to-date record of your CPD how can you demonstrate that you have developed professionally?

British Paramedic Association (BPA) support with CPD

To help you to meet the HPC standards, the College of Paramedics has created the online CPD diary system. This is a simple electronic web-based record that records activities and reflections on learning on an ongoing basis. BPA members are able to access the diary via the BPA website at any time, from anywhere that has internet access.

Standards for CPD

Paramedics must:

- maintain a continuous, up-to-date and accurate record of their CPD activities;
- demonstrate that their CPD activities are a mixture of learning activities relevant to current or future practice;
- seek to ensure that their CPD has contributed to the quality of their practice and service delivery;
- seek to ensure that their CPD benefits the service user; and
- present a written profile containing evidence of their CPD upon request.

(HPC 2006: 12)

HPC Audit

The HPC will carry out its first audit of 2.5 per cent of paramedics in August 2009. This will examine CPD for the registration period August 2007 to August 2009.

If you are selected for audit, the HPC will ask you to complete a CPD profile that summarizes your CPD activities for the period August 2007 to August 2009 (HPC 2006).

Examples of types of CPD activity

This HPC list suggests the kinds of activity that might make up your CPD profile:

Work-based learning

- Analysing significant events
- Case studies
- Clinical audit
- Coaching from others
- Discussions with colleagues
- Evidence of learning activities undertaken as part of your progression on the Knowledge and Skills Framework
- Filling in self-assessment questionnaires
- In-service training
- Involvement in wider work of your employer
- Learning by doing
- Peer review
- Project work or project management
- Reflective practice
- Secondments or job rotation
- Supervising staff or students
- Visiting other departments
- Work shadowing

Professional activity

- Being a national assessor
- Being a tutor
- Being an external examiner
- Being an expert witness
- Being promoted
- Giving presentations at conferences
- Involvement in your professional body
- Lecturing or teaching
- Maintaining or developing specialist skills (for example, musical skills)
- Membership of a specialist interest group
- Mentoring or coaching new staff
- Organizing accredited courses
- Organizing journal clubs or other specialist groups
- Supervising research

Formal/educational

- Attending conferences (Ambex or BPA conference)
- Courses accredited by your professional body
- Distance learning
- Further education
- Going to seminars
- Planning or running a course
- Research and audit
- Writing or editing a chapter in a book
- Writing articles or papers

Self-directed learning

- Keeping a file of your progress
- Reading journals/articles
- Reviewing books or articles
- Updating knowledge through the internet or TV

Other

- Public service
- Voluntary work

If selected, the main parts of your CPD profile will be:

- a summary of your practice history for the last two years (up to 500 words);
- a statement of how you have met our standards of CPD (up to 1500 words); and
- evidence to support your statement.

(Summarized from HPC 2006)

The purpose of each part of the profile

The **summary of your practice history** should help to show the CPD assessors how your CPD activities are linked to your work. This part of the CPD profile should help you to show how your activities are 'relevant to your current or future work'.

Your **statement** of how you have met HPC standards should clearly show how you believe you meet each of the standards, and should refer to all the CPD activities you have undertaken and the **evidence** you are sending in to support your statement.

The **evidence** you send in will show that you have undertaken the CPD activities you have referred to, and should also show how they have improved the quality of your work and benefited service users. Your evidence should include a summary of all your CPD activities. This will show that you meet Standard 1. The CPD assessors should also be able to see how your CPD activities are a mixture of learning activities and are relevant to your work (and therefore meet Standard 2).

Writing the summary of your practice history

Your summary should describe your role and the type of work you do. The summary should identify the people you communicate and work with most and identify the specialist areas you work in, including your main responsibilities, such as your job description if appropriate.

When you have written your statement about how you meet our standards for CPD (see the following explanation), you may find it helpful to go back over your summary of work, to make sure that it clearly explains how your CPD activities are relevant to your future or current work.

Writing your statement

When you write your statement, the HPC expect you to concentrate most on how you meet Standards 3 and 4 – how your CPD activities improve the quality of your work and the benefits to service users.

Suggestions on how you might want to approach writing your statements are listed below.

You could write a statement on how you have updated your knowledge and skills over the last two years, and what learning needs you have met. You may find it helpful to identify three to six points that have contributed to the quality of your work.

These areas will have been identified through your personal development plan (PDP). If you have a PDP, you can provide this as part of your evidence.

Not all paramedics have a PDP or review their role or performance – you may be self-employed, or your employer may not work in this way. But if you do have a personal development plan, you may find it helpful to use this as a starting point for writing your statement. If you do not already have a PDP, you may find it useful to develop one and to use this approach.

Most PDPs involve identifying:

- learning needs;
- learning activities;
- types of evidence; and
- what you have learnt.

CPD and competence

There is no automatic link between your CPD and your competence. This is because it would be possible (although unlikely) for a competent paramedic not to undertake any CPD and yet still meet our standards for their skills and knowledge. Equally, it would be possible for a paramedic who was not competent to complete a lot of CPD activities but still not be fit to practise.

Explanation of how HPC Standards 1–5 can be demonstrated within your CPD profile

Standard 1

You must maintain a continuous, up-to-date and accurate record of your CPD

You can keep a record of your activities in whatever way is most convenient for you. You might choose to keep a folder of papers, perhaps using an online system CPD such as the diary provided by the College of Paramedics on their website (www.Britishparamedic.org).

Your record must be continuous and up-to-date. Your profile will normally concentrate on the CPD you have undertaken in the previous two years.

You will want to fill in your CPD profile honestly and accurately. If you provide false or misleading information in your CPD profile, the HPC will deal with you under their fitness to practise procedures. This could lead to you being struck off the register so that you can no longer practise. Someone who is struck off from the HPC register cannot apply to be registered again for five years.

If you are audited, the HPC will ask you to fill in a form (the CPD profile). This is a form that they will provide you with. In it you must write a statement which tells them how your CPD has met the standards. When you send this in, you must also send in supporting evidence from your personal CPD record.

The simplest way to prove that you have kept a record of your CPD is to send them, as part of your evidence, a summary of all of your CPD activities. This could be in any format you choose, but it is suggested that it might be a simple table which includes the date and 'type' of each activity. See the website of the College of Paramedics BPA.

Standard 2

You must demonstrate that your CPD activities are a mixture of learning activities relevant to current or future practice

You do not need to undertake or log a certain number of hours or days. This is because different people will be able to dedicate different amounts of time to CPD, and also because the time spent on an activity does not necessarily reflect the learning gained from it.

Under this standard, your CPD must include a mixture of learning activities – so you should include different types of learning activity in your CPD record.

Your CPD may be a mixture of what is relevant in your current job, and activities which are helping to prepare you for a future role. Or you may choose to concentrate most or all of your CPD on the new area of work you will be moving into. This means that your CPD may be very different from that which your colleagues undertake, even though you are from the same profession.

If you are managing a team, your CPD may be based around your skills in appraising your team, supporting their development, and financial planning. *It might not even include dealing with patients.*

Standard 3

You must seek to ensure that your CPD has contributed to the quality of your practice and service delivery

You should aim for your CPD to improve the way you work. Your learning activities should lead to you making changes to how you work, which improve the way you provide your service. This may mean that you continue to work as you did before, but you are more confident that you are working effectively.

You do not necessarily have to make drastic changes to how you work to improve the quality of your work and the way you provide your service. You may meet this standard by showing how your work has developed as your skills increase through your learning. In meeting this standard, you should be able to show that your CPD activities are part of your work, contribute to your work, and are not separate from it.

Standard 4

You must seek to ensure that your CPD benefits the service user

Like Standard 3, this standard says that you should 'seek to ensure' (try to make sure). You will meet this standard as long as you have tried to make your CPD benefit service users.

Depending where you work will dictate who are your service users; for many this will be patients. However, if you work in education, your service users may be your students or the team of educationalists you oversee. Similarly, if you work in management, your service users may be your team, or other teams that you are part of. If you work in research, your service users may be the people who use your research. So in this standard, 'service user' means anyone who is primarily affected by your work.

Standard 5

You must present a written profile containing evidence of your CPD upon request

If you are chosen for audit, the HPC will send you a CPD profile. Under this standard, you must fill the profile in, with details of how you have met the standards for CPD. You must return the profile to them, with evidence to support it, by the deadline set.

It is believed that CPD can and does take many forms, and that it should not set down exactly how paramedics should learn. It is also believed that paramedics may already be taking part in activities through which they learn, and which develop their work, but they may not call these activities CPD.

Many people think of CPD as only being formal education (for example, going on courses). The HPC standards take account of the fact that a course may not be the most useful kind of CPD for all health professionals, and some health professionals may not have access to courses, or are unable to gain funding support or study time. Different registrants will have different development needs, and their CPD activities may be very different.

Registrant working in a clinical role

- Attending a short course on new laws affecting your work
- Appraising an article with a group of colleagues
- Giving colleagues a presentation on a new technique

Registrant working in education

- Member of a learning and teaching committee
- Review for a professional journal
- Studying for a formal teaching award

Registrant working in management

- Member of an occupational group for managers
- Studying management modules
- Supporting the development and introduction of a national or local policy

Registrant involved in research

- Presentation at a conference
- Member of a local ethics research committee
- Articles for scientific journals

Two years' registration

The HPC will only audit registrants who have been registered for more than two years (HPC 2006). They believe that all registrants should undertake CPD throughout their careers; they also believe that registrants should be allowed at least two years on the register to build up evidence of their CPD activities before they are audited.

This means that if you are a recent graduate, and you renew your registration for the first time, you will not be chosen for audit. Similarly, if you have had a break from work, and you have just come back onto the register, you will not be chosen for audit the first time you renew your registration.

What happens to your completed CPD profile?

The HPC will ask CPD assessors to assess your CPD profile. At least one of these assessors will be a paramedic.

While your profile is being assessed, and during any appeal that takes place, you will stay on the register and can continue to work.

There are three possible outcomes at this point.

- Your profile meets the standards – you will stay on the register. They will write to you and let you know.
- More information is needed – they will write to you and let you know what information the assessors need to decide whether you meet the standards of CPD. You will stay on the register while you send more information to the assessors.
- Your profile does not meet the standards – the CPD assessors will then decide whether to offer you an extra three months to meet the standards of CPD or to recommend that your registration should end.

The CPD assessors will decide whether to offer you an extra three months by considering whether:

- you appear to have filled in your CPD profile honestly and accurately;
- you have met any or some of the standards; and
- within the three months, it would be possible for you to undertake CPD which would meet the standards.

Finding out more

Published example profiles can be seen on the HPC website (www.hpc-uk.org). These profiles, which were put together in partnership with the College of Paramedics, are intended to show how health professionals can show that their CPD activities have met these standards, and how they can write a statement that shows this.

For even more information about the CPD audit, read the HPC document *Continuing Professional Development and Your Registration*. This is a helpful document, with more detail about continuing professional development, and about the audit process. You can download this document from the HPC website or you can write to the HPC to ask for a copy.

Conclusion

CPD is now formally recognized as an important part of being registered. This has given professional bodies and organizations the opportunity to campaign for greater support and recognition of your CPD activities, from your employers and other organizations. The consultation document and subsequent recommendations for continuing professional development was signed in February 2007 by 11 professional bodies representing health professionals, including the College of Paramedics British Paramedic Association. Mandatory continuing professional development for paramedics is currently six days (45 hours) per year, to be evidenced in the ways discussed earlier in the chapter.

Chapter key points

- Explanation of the role and value of continuing professional development (CPD).
- The role of the Health Professions Council in CPD and discussion of the relevant standards of proficiency.
- The chapter provides examples of CPD activity for inclusion in your profile.
- Each of the relevant standards are discussed and ideas are provided about how you can meet the standards within your written profile.
- An explanation of what will happen to your completed profile is given along with advice about how to obtain further information and guidance.

References suggested reading

Brookes, N. (2003) *Standards of Conduct, Performance and Ethics. Your Duties as a Registrant.* London: Health Professions Council.

Health Professions Council/Allied Health Professions Project (2002) *Demonstrating Competence through CPD.* London: HPC.

Health Professions Council (2003a) *Standards of Proficiency: Paramedics.* London: HPC.

Health Professions Council (2003b) *Standards of Conduct, Performance and Ethics.* London: HPC.

Health Professions Council (2006) *Your Guide to Our Standards for Continuing Professional Development.* London: HPC.

Useful websites

College of Paramedics/British Paramedic Association: www.Britishparamedic.org
Health Professions Council: www.hpc-uk.org

Conclusion

This book has provided an introduction to many subjects relevant to paramedic practice; some can be broadly categorized within the social science genre. These subjects are included within a foundation degree or undergraduate paramedic science higher education programme. The main aim has been to provide a foundation upon which students can plan their future study or further investigation. Further reading and study will be required, to gain a more in-depth understanding of any of the included subjects.

The book has provided a clear overview of the many theoretical aspects relevant to paramedic practice in the twenty-first century, in addition to the more practical aspects of the role. An understanding and appreciation of the importance of all the subject areas contained within the book will equip the twenty-first-century higher education-educated paramedic with a holistic and informed view of their patients and families.

The editor and contributors are passionate about their subject areas and regularly teach these subjects to healthcare professionals. Our ultimate aim is to raise the standard of holisitic care given to patients and their families.

Index